ABDOMINAL SURGERY

Edited by **Fethi Derbel**

Abdominal Surgery
http://dx.doi.org/10.5772/3020
Edited by Fethi Derbel

Contributors
Fethi Derbel, Nadia Mama, Hela Jemni, Nadia Arifa Achour, Ould Chavey Sidiya, Kaled Kadri, Mehdi Gaha, Ibtisem Hasni, Kalthoum Tlili, Aysin Alagol, Jens Børglum, Kenneth Jensen, Ignacio Ferrón-Celma, Carmen Olmedo, Alfonso Mansilla, Ana Garcia-Navarro, Karim Muffak, Pablo Bueno, Jose-Antonio Ferrón, Mohamed Ben Mabrouk, Mehdi Ben Hadj Hamida, Jaafar Mazhoud, Sabri Youssef, Ali Ben Ali, Hasni Ibtissem, Arifa Nadia, Chedia El Ouni, Walid Naija, Moncef Mokni, Ridha Ben Hadj Hamida, Enrico Maria Pasqual, Serena Bertozzi

Published by InTech
Janeza Trdine 9, 51000 Rijeka, Croatia

Publishing Process Manager Romina Skomersic
Technical Editor InTech Prepress, Novi Sad
Cover InTech Design team

Additional hard copies can be obtained from orders@intechopen.com

Abdominal Surgery, Edited by Fethi Derbel
p. cm.
ISBN 978-953-51-0691-3

Meet the editor

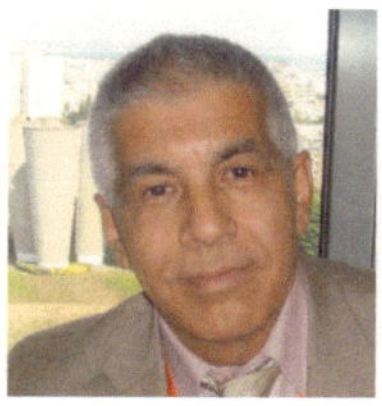

Professor Fethi Derbel was born in 1960, in Tunisia. He received his medical degree from the Sousse Faculty of Medicine at Sousse, Tunisia. He completed his surgical residency in General Surgery at University Hospital Farhat Hached of Sousse and was a member of Unit of Liver Transplantation in the University of Rennes, France. Professor Derbel is presently working at the department of surgery in Sahloul Hospital, Sousse. His hospital activities are mostly concerned with laparoscopic, colorectal, pancreatic, hepato-biliary and gastric surgery. He is also a professor at the school of Medicine in Djibouti, past member of the medical committee at the University Hospital Sahloul, Sousse and member of the National College of Surgeons in Tunisia. Professor Derbel has published many articles in journals and collaborates intensively with InTech Open Access Publisher as an editor.

Contents

Preface

We are very pleased to provide you with this book dealing with abdominal surgery.

The chapters in this book are written by surgeons, radiologists, anesthesiologists and oncologists from different hospitals in Tunisia, Turkey, Denmark, Spain and Italy. Together with basic surgical principles, the unique local experiences and perspectives are presented.

The present book is subdivided into three sections and six chapters:

1. Abdominal Trauma imaging
2. Anesthetic Management of Abdominal Surgery
3. Advances in the use of ultrasound-guided truncal blocks for perioperative pain management
4. Study of vitamin C administration effect on postoperative plasma IL concentrations in septic patients after abdominal surgery
5. Hydatid cysts of the liver: Diagnosis, complications and treatment
6. Abdominal advanced oncologic surgery

Most radiologists are frequently confronted with trauma patients in their everyday practice. It is of vital importance that the radiologist should assume full responsibility with the trauma team responsible for managing the patient to ensure that a rapid and optimal diagnosis is made.

The chapter about the abdominal trauma imaging provides a very comprehensive and integrated overview on modern imaging protocols and minimally invasive treatment options in the pelvic trauma. It also underlines the importance of computed tomography imaging in blunt abdominal trauma and the role of interventional radiology in acute haemorrhage. The chapter will be a useful aid to medical students, radiologists, surgical trainees, physicians and emergency doctors who wish to gain a greater understanding of abdominal and pelvic imaging and how it can improve their clinical practice. Radiology trainees will also find this a helpful "aide-mémoire" to consolidate their knowledge.

I would like to congratulate professor Hela Gharbi Jemni, Nadia Mama Larbi, Nadia Arifa Achour, khaled Kadri, Kalthoum Graiess Tlili and the team of Radiology at Sahloul Hospital on the superb work and illustrations of this chapter.

I highly recommend this chapter to all radiologists involved in the management of abdominal trauma patients and to trauma surgeons and intensive care physicians.

Anesthesia is a medical treatment which leads human body to abnormal condition. This means that anesthetic management is always accompanied by risks of accidental events, and "vigilance" is considered as the most important duty of anesthesiologists.

The importance of the anesthetist in perioperative care cannot be too greatly emphasized. Correct patient selection and procedure planning can only be optimized by a team approach and together with the surgeon; the anesthetist forms the core of the team. A thorough understanding of the underlying physiology of the gastrointestinal tract is important and a logical starting place for this book.

Two chapters in this book "Anesthetic Management of Abdominal Surgery" and "Advances in the Use of Ultrasound-Guided Truncal Blocks for Perioperative Pain Management" give answers to different questions concerning the field of anesthesiology and the treatment of the perioperative pain in abdominal surgery. A very interesting prospective study about **vitamin C administration effect on postoperative plasma IL-6 concentrations in septic patients after abdominal surgery was carried out and shows very interesting results.**

Surgery continues to evolve as new technology, techniques, and knowledge are incorporated into the care of surgical patients. There are two surgical chapters in the book - the first concerns the hydatid disease of the liver, and the second concerns the Abdominal advanced oncologic surgery.

Although this book does not cover all the aspects related to the abdominal surgery, it is intended for at least two kinds of readers:

a. Residents of intermediate and advanced courses in medicine;
b. Anesthesiologists, oncologists, surgeons, radiologists and all doctors whatever the specialty.

As editor in chief of this book, I would like to acknowledge the efforts made by all of the contributing authors and the entire editorial team in the publishing of this book especially Ms Romina Skomersic for her very precious collaboration. Their dedication to the publication of the most contemporary and comprehensive scientific data has resulted with this excellent work. I would like to dedicate this book to all my colleagues - surgeons, pathologists, oncologists, radiologists and anethesists at Sahloul hospital. I also dedicate it especially to Professor Ridha Ben Hadj Hamida, surgeon at the department of surgery in Sousse. A special dedication to my colleagues Jaafar Mazhoud, Mohamed Ben Mabrouk, Mahdi Ben Haj Hamida , Sabri Youssef, Ibtissam Hasni and Moncef Mokni for their contribution in this book, and Mr Fayçal Mansouri, the president of the university of Sousse.

I would also acknowledge Mr Bouraoui El Weslati professor of English at Tark Ibn Zied School in Sousse for his great help in revising the manuscript.

The main person I want to thank is my wonderful wife, Elhem, who regularly reassured me that I could pull this off. I also thank my daughter Rania, and sons Raed and Nader who were always proud. All my best wishes go to my mother Jamila to whom I wish a quick recovery.

Finally, I thank the authors of these excellent articles. They were willing to share their knowledge with a wider audience and to do so for no fee. I enjoyed working with them, getting to know them, and learning from them. I apologize to those friends whose names I may have overlooked.

Fethi Derbel
Professor of General and Digestive Surgery
University Hospital Sahloul
Sousse
Tunisia

Section 1

Role of Imaging in Exploration of the Abdomen

Chapter 1

Abdominal Trauma Imaging

Nadia Mama, Hela Jemni, Nadia Arifa Achour, Ould Chavey Sidiya,
Kaled Kadri, Mehdi Gaha, Ibtisem Hasni and Kalthoum Tlili

Additional information is available at the end of the chapter

http://dx.doi.org/10.5772/50426

1. Introduction

Isolated blunt abdominal trauma (BAT) represents about 5% of annual trauma mortality from blunt trauma. As part of multiple-site injury (polytrauma), BAT contributes another 15% of trauma mortality. In the abdominal trauma, the best exploration strategy is one that leads most quickly and reliably in the diagnosis of surgical injury. This strategy must be established based on hemodynamic status and clinical guidance but should never delay a therapeutic homeostasis. Early recognition and treatment decisions have been greatly impacted by increasingly sophisticated cross-sectional imaging and image-guided, minimally invasive therapies.

2. Imaging techniques

2.1. Plain radiographs

Plain x-ray plays a limited role in the evaluation of blunt abdominal trauma. Abdominal radiographs are usually unnecessary. X-rays of the chest and pelvis are often obtained to evaluate for concurrent thoracic or pelvic injuries. Abnormal chest x-ray findings of pneumothorax and rib fractures are associated with intraabdominal injuries and are indications for abdominal imaging if a mechanism for multisystem trauma is present. Common findings include free abdominal air (pneumoperitoneum), pneumothorax, and hemothorax. In the case of gunshot wounds, x-rays identify the location and number of retained projectiles.

2.2. Ultrasound

Ultrasound has become a common part of the initial assessment of blunt abdominal trauma. Ultrasound serves a screening function because it assesses for the presence of free fluid in the abdomen or pericardium but does not explicitly identify the source. The focused assessment with sonography in trauma (FAST) examination has been a standard part of the diagnostic algorithm since the 1990s in most U.S. trauma centers. The FAST exam looks for intra peritoneal and intra pericardial anechoic material representing fluid—which in the setting of trauma is assumed to be blood.

Advantages of ultrasound include portability (allowing it to be used during resuscitation), lack of ionizing radiation exposure, repeatability (allowing evaluation of changes in patient condition), and rapidity of the exam. Disadvantages include significant operator dependence and low sensitivity according detection of solid organ injury.

Ultrasound is considered most useful in detection of solid organ injuries with associated hemoperitoneum. It is considered insensitive for the detection of bowel or retroperitoneal injuries.

However, a recent study of Moriwaki and al **[1]** found ultrasound was 85% sensitive and 100% specific for detection of free air in a prospective study of 484 patients. Some small studies have also investigated the utility of ultrasound contrast agents to detect active bleeding **[2]**. Ultrasound is relatively sensitive for free abdominal fluid. In a study, continuous scanning of Morison's pouch during infusion of DPL fluid revealed a mean detection limit of 619 mL. Only 10% of ultrasonographers (attending physicians and residents in emergency medicine, radiology, and surgery) detected volumes less than 400 mL. The sensitivity at 1 L was 97% [3]. Ultrasound is not sufficiently sensitive to exclude intraabdominal injury, limiting its utility as a definitive test for abdominal trauma. It allows selection of patients for CT and follow up.

2.3. Computed tomography in trauma

For most stable trauma patients, CT has become the definitive imaging modality of choice when intraabdominal injury is suspected. CT is rapid and highly sensitive and specific for many important injury types. The information provided by CT allows prognosis of injury and selective nonoperative management in both blunt and penetrating trauma. CT is less sensitive for some important injuries, including bowel and diaphragmatic trauma, a limitation that must be recognized to prevent clinical errors following a negative CT. For the evaluation of blunt abdominal or flank trauma, intravenous (IV) contrast should be routinely used, but oral contrast should not. We use 150 mL of intravenous contrast, infused at 2-4 mL per second, with CT being performed after a 60 second delay. A prior acquisition without intravenous contrast is recommended. It assesses solid organ hematomas and sentinel hematoma. Arterial acquisition is performed when chest exploration is indicated. Delayed acquisition (2-3 minutes) is performed when renal lesions or active bleeding are diagnosed. A number of studies have evaluated the safety and sensitivity of the triple-contrast CT approach. A metaanalysis performed by Goodman and al. **[4]**, performed to determine the predictive value of CT for laparotomy in hemodynamically stable patients with penetrating abdominal trauma. They identified 180 studies but included only 5 because of methodologic concerns. The pooled sensitivity, specificity, negative predictive value, positive predictive value, and accuracy were 94.90%, 95.38%, 98.62%, 84.51%, and 94.70%, respectively.

Overall, triple-contrast CT appears to be a safe management strategy in highly selected stable patients without peritonitis on examination. Multiple studies have demonstrated the possibility of missed diaphragmatic injuries and, rarely, missed operative bowel injuries. Following a negative triple-contrast CT, observation or close follow-up should be ensured.

3. Lesional spectrum

3.1. Hemoperitoneum

Fluid is anechoic (black) on ultrasound. In the case of small amounts of hemoperitoneum, fluid may be visible only as an anechoic stripe separating the liver and the kidney on the right, or the spleen and the kidney on the left. Fluid may also accumulate between the spleen and diaphragm. Free fluid pooled in the pelvis is visible as anechoic collections lateral to the bladder on a transverse view. Free fluid may also be visible in the recto uterine recess (pouch of Douglas) in females using a sagittal view. In cases of gross hemoperitoneum, loops of bowel may be seen floating in blood.

Traumatic hemoperitoneum may be detected at CT anywhere in the peritoneal cavity.

Measuring the CT attenuation of intraperitoneal fluid (**figures 1, 2.**) has proved exceedingly useful in its characterization, because intraperitoneal fluid collections in trauma patients may not always represent blood. Although there is variation with individual scanners, hemoperitoneum usually measures greater than 30 HU. By comparison, water-dense fluids in a trauma patient, such as ascites, urine, bile, or intestinal contents, measure 0 to 5 or 10 HU.

The recognition of water-dense fluids can be assisted by visual comparison with a fluid-filled structure, such as the gallbladder, or the soft tissue density of abdominal wall musculature; however, one may be misled by appearance only.

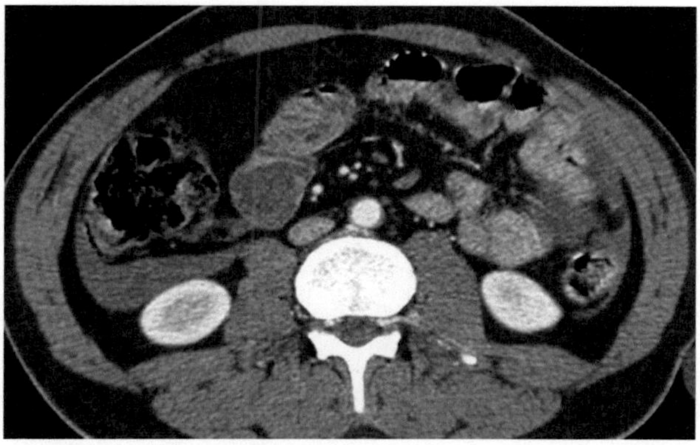

Figure 1. Axial contrast-enhanced CT images show hemoperitoneum: free fluid that has higher densities than gastric contents on CT soft-tissue windows. Intraperitoneal fluid is located in paracolic gutters and especially in perisplenic regions. Note that in the latter location hemoperitoneum have high density related to a splenic injury.

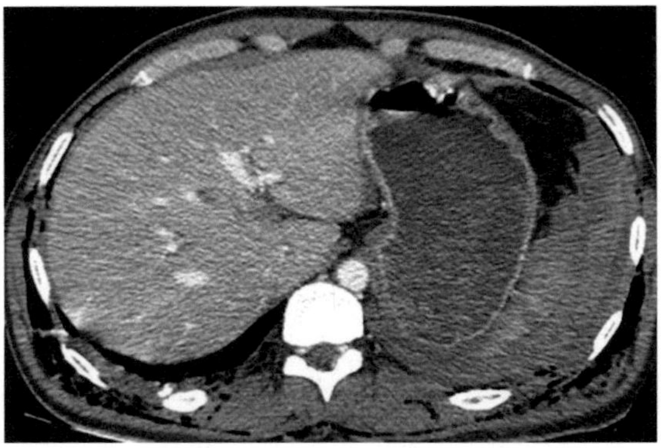

Figure 2. Axial contrast-enhanced CT images show hemoperitoneum: free fluid that has higher densities than gastric contents on CT soft-tissue windows. Intraperitoneal fluid is located in paracolic gutters and especially in perisplenic regions. Note that in the latter location hemoperitoneum have high density related to a splenic injury.

3.2. Pneumoperitoneum

Pneumoperitoneum is rare following blunt abdominal injury but can indicate bowel perforation. Soft-tissue windows are used at first, they can detect large amounts of Pneumoperitoneum who appear black **(Figure 3.)**. Smaller collections are attempted on lung windows, followed by bone windows. When detected on CT, it is not specific for bowel injury because air tracking from thoracic injuries can collect in the abdomen. Following penetrating abdominal injury, Pneumoperitoneum detected on CT is likely to indicate bowel perforation and prompts laparotomy in most cases.

Pneumoperitoneum is also sometimes visible on ultrasound. Air is hyperechoic and disrupts the ultrasound beam, preventing visualization of deeper structures. Because bowel gas is normally present in the anterior midline abdomen, free air should be sought overlying the liver, where air is not normally present.

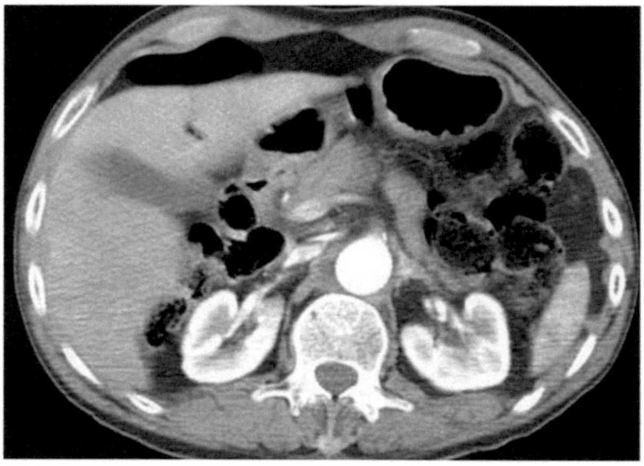

Figure 3. Axial contrast-enhanced CT image shows free air next to the anterior face of the liver: low attenuation on abdominal window. This pneumoperitoneum is related to a post traumatic colonic injury.

3.3. Active bleeding

With the injection of contrast, active bleeding is visible as a bright white "blush" or amorphous collection on arterial phase imaging within a hypodense injured solid organ indicates active bleeding. This must be distinguished from normal enhancement of vessels within solid organs, such as portal and hepatic vessels within the liver. On delayed imaging the area of active extravasation remains high in attenuation and increases in size **(Figure 4.)**, a result of ongoing bleeding from the injured vessel after the initial phases of scanning.

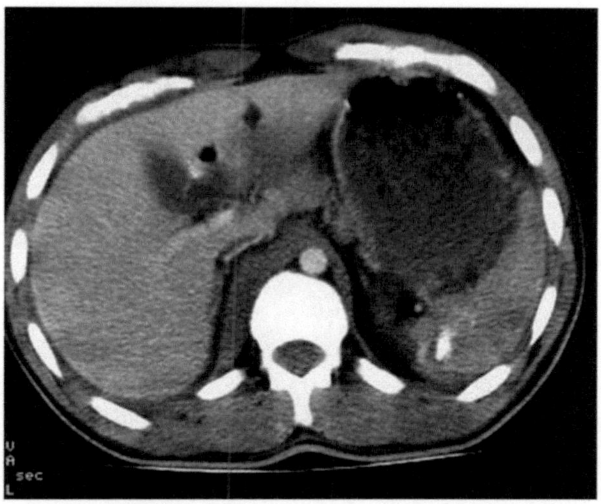

Figure 4. Contrast enhanced CT scan: spleen injury: active contrast extravasation reflecting active bleeding

3.4. Lacerations

The laceration may initially be difficult to recognize in sonography or may appear slightly echogenic band. Acute splenic lacerations are seen on contrast-enhanced MDCT as linear or branching areas of low attenuation with well-defined margins **(Figure 5.)**. When lacerations extend through the organ capsule, hemoperitoneum results; if the capsule is intact, a subcapsular hematoma may be demonstrated. With time, the lacerations decrease in size and number. The margins become less well defined, and the area becomes isodense compared with normal splenic parenchyma. Although healing changes may be seen within 2 to 3 days, complete resolution may take weeks to months, depending on the size of the original injury. An increase in the number of lacerations on follow-up MDCT should alert the radiologist to the possibility of injury progression, and close clinical follow-up with MDCT or angiography is advised. Splenic clefts may mimic lacerations on MDCT but typically have smooth or rounded margins. Fat may be periphery and become less visible, splenic clefts remain unchanged in appearance on delayed images.

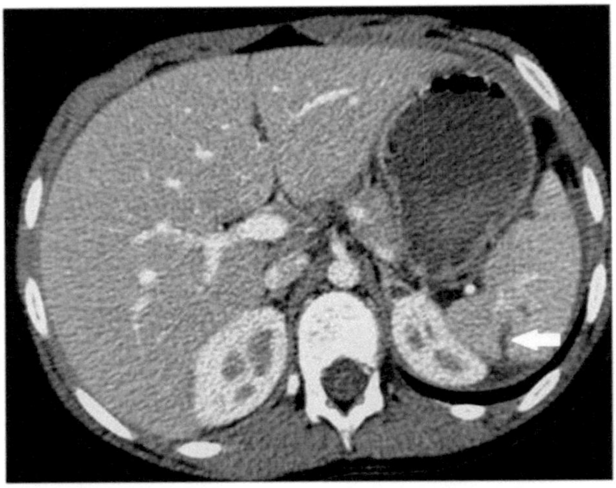

Figure 5. Contrast enhanced CT scan: small splenic laceration that does not involve the hilum with free fluid surrounding the spleen

3.5. Contusions

They represent areas of injury. They appear on contrast-enhanced CT as parenchymal areas of low attenuation with irregular edges **(Figure 6.)**. Contusions are invariably a minor injury and gradually decrease in size as the injury heals.

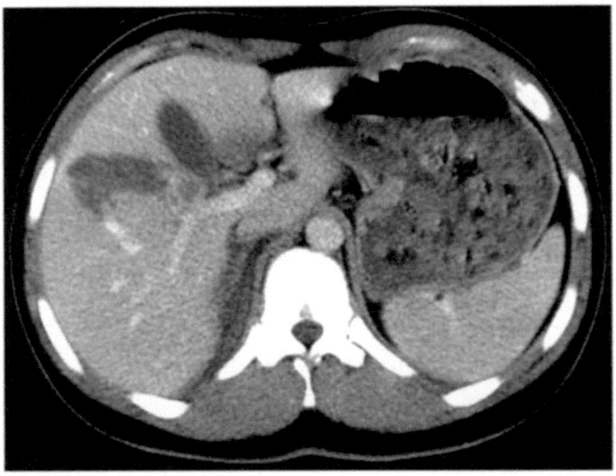

Figure 6. Contrast-enhanced CT scan showing an hypodense area on the liver relevant to a hepatic contusion

3.6. Fractures

- When the bands of laceration cross the hypodense parenchyma, joining two opposite edges through the hilum, they are called fracture **(Figures 7., 8.)**.

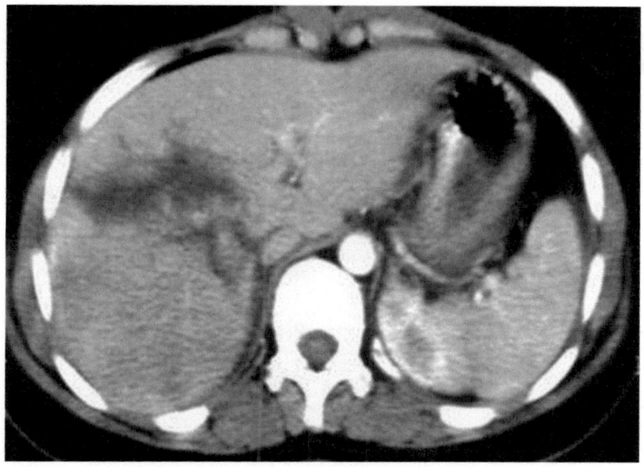

Figure 7. Contrast-enhanced CT scan showing a complex hepatic lacerations : hepatic fracture

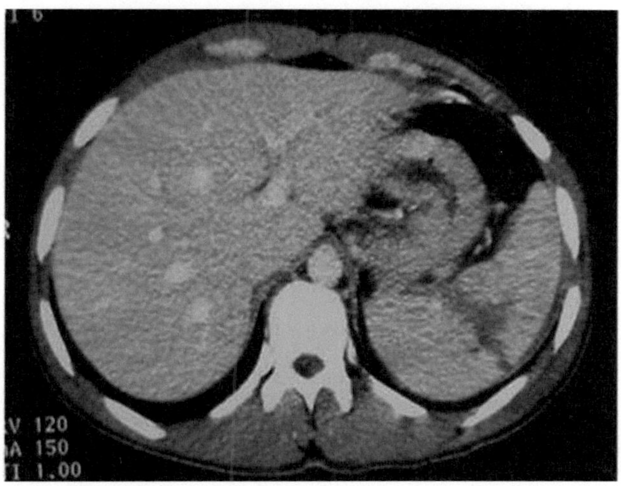

Figure 8. Contrast-enhanced CT scan : linear hypodensity crossing the splenic thickness: splenic fracture. Note free fluid surrounding the spleen.

3.7. Hematoma

- **Subcapsular hematomas:** appear as crescentic regions of hyperdensity compared with adjacent normal parenchyma. After contrast administration, subcapsular hematomas are seen as a low-attenuation collection between the splenic capsule and enhancing splenic parenchyma that compress the underlying contrast-opacified organ parenchyma **(Figure 9.)**. This finding is useful in differentiating subcapsular hematomas from free intraperitoneal fluid or blood. In sonography, it appears as a hyperechoic or hypoechoic rim or crescent
- **Intraparenchymatic hematomas:** appear as a round hyperdensity compared with adjacent normal parenchyma. After contrast administration, they appear as low-attenuation zones within the parenchyma; these may be homogeneous or

inhomogeneous **(Figure 10.)**. On sonography, they are present as a localized area of increased echogenicity **(Figures 11., 12., 13.)**.

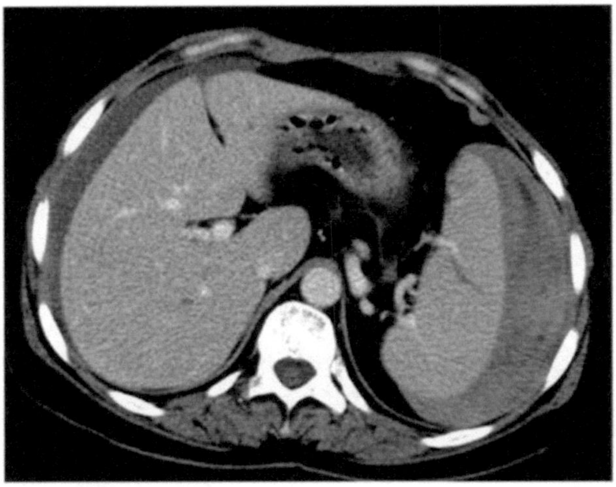

Figure 9. Contrast-enhanced CT scan : sub capsular splenic hematoma that involves more than 50% of surface area

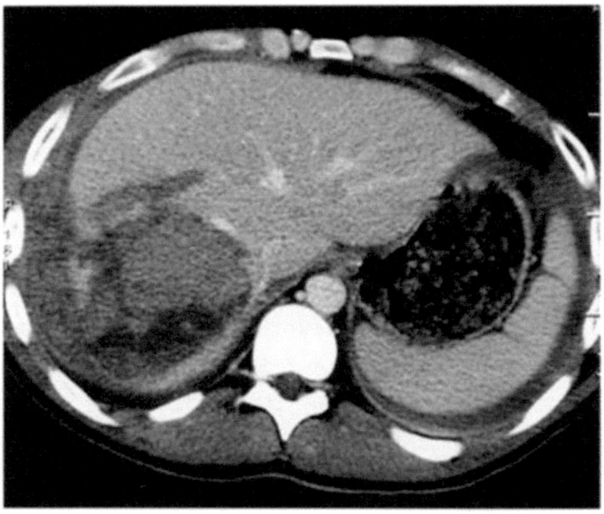

Figure 10. Contrast-enhanced CT scan : multiple lacerations and a parenchymal hematoma. Note abundant hemoperitoneum.

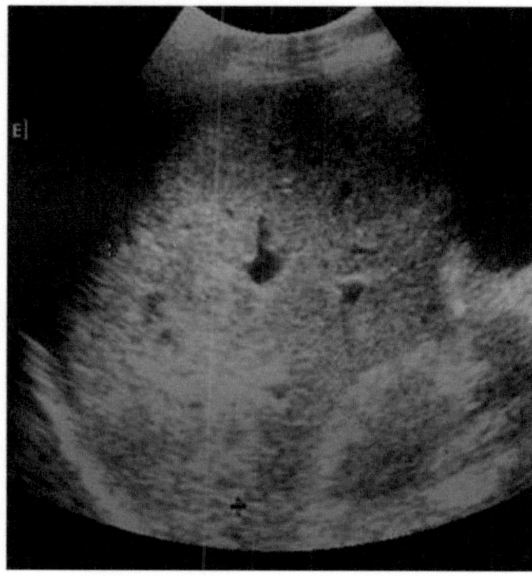

Figure 11. Ultrasonographic evolution of a hepatic contusion: Hyperechoic post traumatic area in the liver consistent with a hematoma.

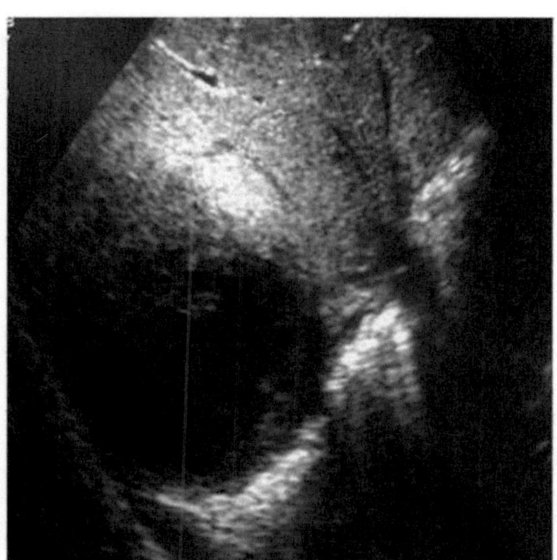

Figure 12. Ultrasonographic evolution of a hepatic contusion: US at the third day after trauma: hematoma liquefaction.

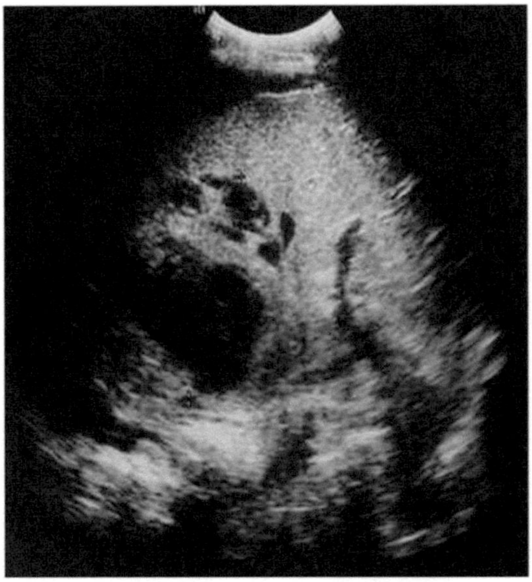

Figure 13. Ultrasonographic evolution of a hepatic contusion: US at the seventh day: decrease in the size of the hematoma.

3.8. IVC shock

In cases of severe volume depletion (generally from hemorrhagic shock following trauma), the infrahepatic **inferior vena cava (IVC)** appears flattened. This appearance can occur in patients before the development of clinical hypotension or hemodynamic collapse and demands immediate volume resuscitation **(figure 14.)**.

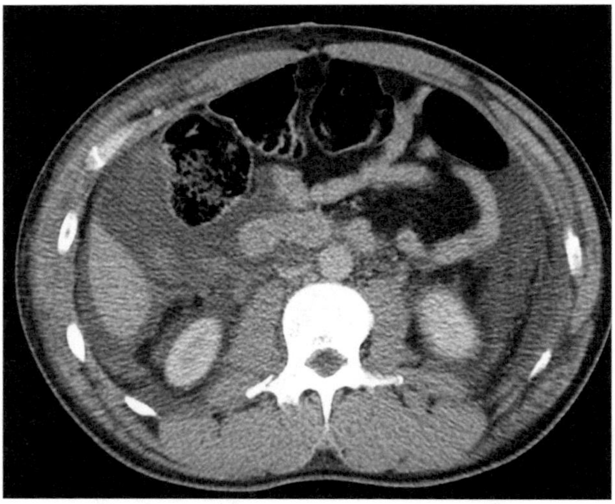

Figure 14. Contrast-enhanced CT scan : flattened IVC related to hemodynamic collapse

Shock bowel is a term for secondary bowel injury resulting from sustained systemic hypotension. The CT appearance includes *diffuse* bowel wall thickening visible on CT.

CT hypotension complex associates multiple findings: Shock bowel with IVC and aortic flattening, abnormal pancreatic enhancement and peripancreatic fluid, and poor enhancement of the spleen and liver because of hypotension.

4. Spleen injury

The spleen is the intra-abdominal organ most often injured as a result of blunt trauma. The spleen is the most vascular organ of the body and, for this reason, splenic injury is potentially life threatening. The most common mechanism for such injury is motor vehicle collision. Left lower rib fractures are suggestive of spleen injury, although an intact rib cage does not exclude spleen trauma. The other trauma mechanisms are penetrating trauma stab, iatrogenic trauma following colonoscopy and spontaneous spleen rupture in some diseases that involve the spleen like infectious mononucleosis, hemopathies or metastasis. Nonsurgical management is becoming the preferred treatment method for adult patients (with blunt splenic injuries) who are hemodynamically stable **[5]**.

Ultrasonography is a quick and noninvasive technique for detecting intra-abdominal blood. When hemoperitoneum is present and mainly when it is peri splenic, it highly suggests spleen trauma. However, a high number of significant abdominal organ injuries occur without associated hemoperitoneum. A large retrospective study performed at the University of Maryland Shock Trauma Center (UMSTC) showed that 57 (27%) of 210 splenic injuries were found to have no hemoperitoneum on admission computed tomography (CT) **[6]**. The Doppler color does not improve US performances. Contrast enhanced ultrasound seems to be a promising technique. MDCT is highly accurate (98%) in diagnosing splenic injury **[7]**. It is important to image for splenic injury during the portal-venous phase, because heterogeneous enhancement in the early arterial phase may simulate injury. The arterial phase is useful in differentiating between active arterial bleeding and posttraumatic vascular injuries, including pseudoaneurysm and traumatic arteriovenous fistulae. The principle types of splenic injury include hematoma, laceration, active hemorrhage, posttraumatic splenic infarct, and vascular injuries, including posttraumatic pseudoaneurysms and arteriovenous fistulae **[8], (figures 5., 8., 15., 16., 17. 18., 19.)**.

Spleen injuries are graded in severity based on CT appearance using a five-point scale **(Table1.)** according to AAST scaling **[9, 10, 11]**. Grading of splenic trauma serves many purposes, even if it cannot reliably be used as a prognostic indicator when nonoperative management is chosen. Marmery et al. state, "The purpose of a grading system is to standardize reporting, plan appropriate management, and enable comparisons between institutions and studies **[11]**. We must note that the presence of splenic vascular injuries is a predictor of failure of nonoperative management that is not explicitly defined under the 1987 original or 1994 revised AAST splenic trauma grading system; Marmery et al. promote their alternative grading system in which vascular splenic injuries are better defined **(table2)**.

Spleen	Injury type	Description of injury	AIS
I	Hematoma	Subscapular, <10 % surface area	2
	laceration	Capsular tear < 1 cm parenchymental depth	2
II	Hematoma	Subscapular, 10 to 50 % surface area intraparenchymaental < 5 cm in diameter	2
	laceration	Capsular tear, 1 to 3 cm parenchymental depth, that does not involve a trabecular vessel.	2
III	Hematoma	Subscapular, > 50 % surface area or expending; ruptured subscapular or parenchymental hematoma; intraparenchymental hematoma> 5 cm or expending.	3
	laceration	> 3 cm parenchymental depth or involve a trabecular vessel.	3
IV	laceration	Laceration involving segmental or hilar vessels producing major devascularization (> 25 % of spleen)	4
V	hematome	Completely shattered spleen	5
	laceration	Hilar vascular injury devascularizes spleen	5

Table 1. Alternate grading system for splenic trauma **[11]**.

Grade		criteria
1		Subscapular hematoma < 1cm thick Laceration < 1cm parenchymal depth Parenchymal hematoma < 1cm diameter
2		Subscapular hematoma 1-3 cm thick Laceration 1-3 cm parenchymal depth Parenchymal hematoma 1-3 cm diameter
3		Splenic capsular disruption Subscapular hematoma >3 cm thick Laceration >3 cm parenchymal depth Parenchymal hematoma >3 cm diameter
4	4a	Active intraparenchymal and subcapsular bleeding Splenic vascular injury (pseudoaneurysm or arteriovenous fistula) Shattered spleen
	4b	Active intra peritoneal bleeding

Table 2. Alternate grading system for splenic trauma in which vascular injuries are better defined **[11]**.

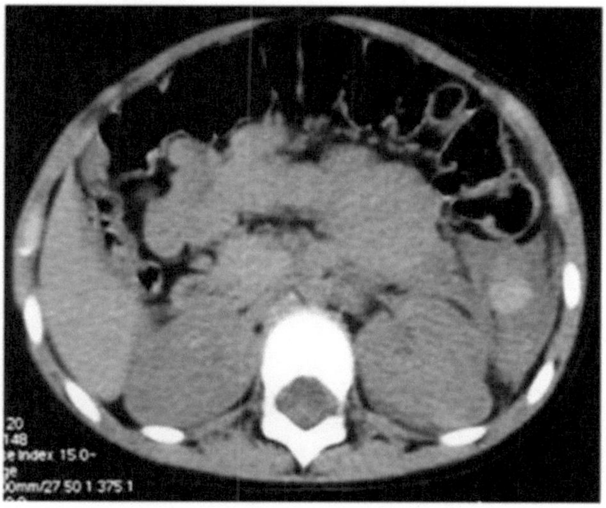

Figure 15. Contrast-unenhanced CT scan: Localized collection of clotted blood : the sentinel clot.

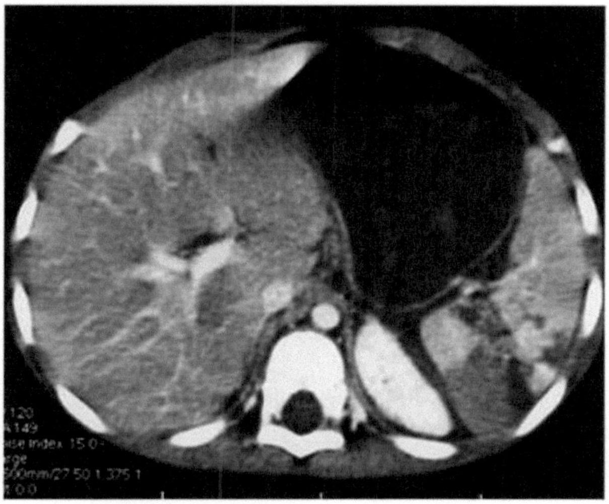

Figure 16. Same patient: Contrast-enhanced CT scan: multiple splenic lacerations. The sentinel clot is indicating the location of the injury.

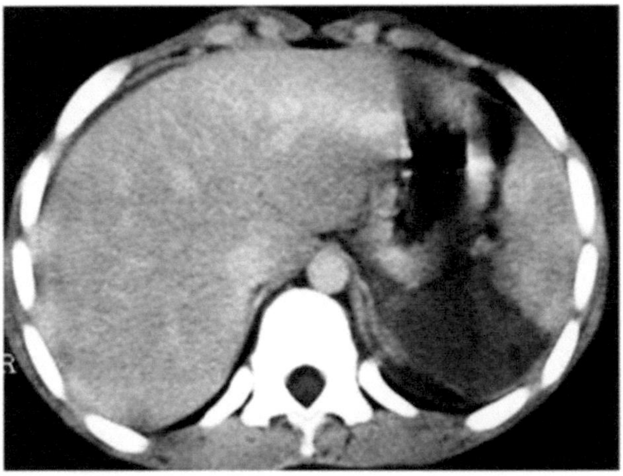

Figure 17. Grade IV AAST splenic injury : segmental devascularization involving more than 50% of the spleen

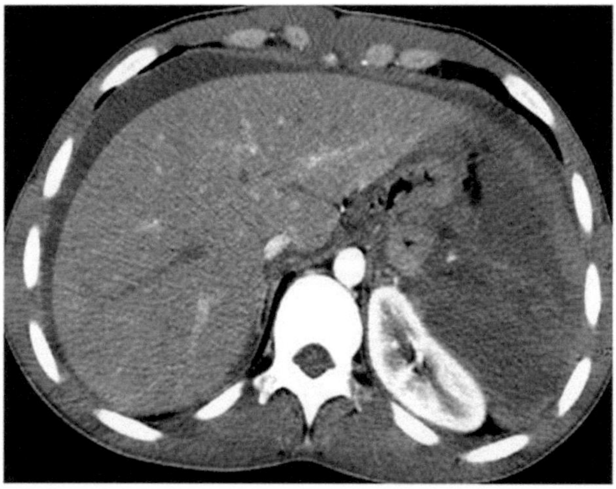

Figure 18. Grade V AAST splenic injury: complete splenic devascularization

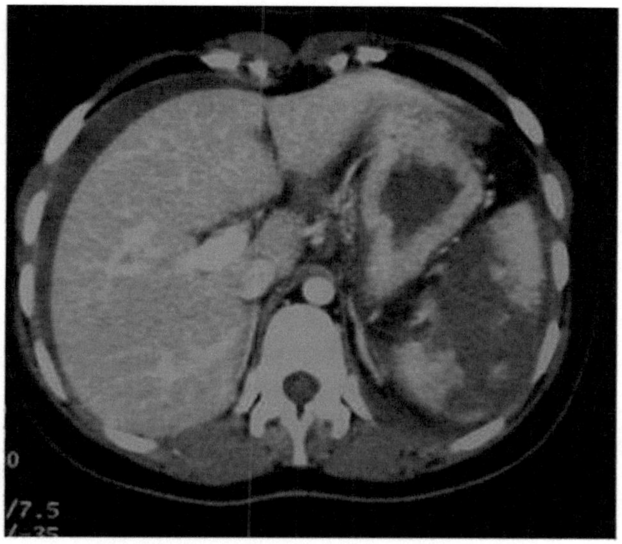

Figure 19. Grade V AAST splenic injury : Completely shattered spleen

5. Liver injury

The liver is frequently injured in blunt trauma. The prevalence of liver injury in patients who have sustained blunt multiple trauma has been reported to be 1%–8% **[12]**. However, liver injuries can be detected in up to 25% of patients with blunt trauma if whole-body computed tomography (CT) is performed as the initial diagnostic procedure in severely injured patients admitted to the trauma center. Isolated hepatic lesions are rare and in 77–90% of cases, lesions of other organs and viscera are involved **[13]**. Blunt liver trauma still carries a significant morbidity and mortality. The reported mortality rate attributable to blunt liver injury ranges from 4.1% to 11.7% **[12, 14, 15]**.

Detected lesions are the consequence of 3 different mechanisms: sudden deceleration such as in crash-car events, direct impact or penetrating wound. The more involved site is the right lobe, posterior–superior segments particularly, because it is the more voluminous portion of the liver; posterior superior hepatic segments are proximal to fixed anatomical structures such as ribs and spine, that may have an important role in producing the lesion. Coronal ligamentous insertion in this region increases the effect of the acceleration–deceleration mechanism. Associated lesions usually are homolateral costal fractures, lesions of the inferior right pulmonary lobe, haemothorax, pneumothorax, renal and/or adrenal lesions **[16]**.

Traumatic lesions of the left hepatic lobe are rare and usually associated with direct impact of the superior abdomen. Associated lesions with left hepatic lobe injuries include sternal fractures, pancreatic, myocardial, duodenal and transverse colon lesions **[16]**. Lesions of the caudate lobe are extremely rare, usually not isolated and are found with other significant lesions.

Generally, hemodynamically stable patients are submitted to sonographic examination for detection of fluid collections and, possibly, of parenchymal lesions. Sonographic findings of a traumatic lesion or of peritoneal fluid are an indication for CT examination. Patients in critical clinical condition go directly to CT examination of the abdomen and pelvis. CT with IV contrast is highly sensitive for liver injuries.

As reported in literature **[9, 17, 18]**.

Radiological findings of traumatic lesion of the liver are: lacerations **(Figure 20.)**, contusions, subcapsular/central hematoma, active hemorrhage **(figure 10., figure 21.)**, periportal tracking **(Figure 22.)**, juxtahepatic venous injuries and avulsion of the hepatic pedicle.

Hepatic lacerations are the most common type of parenchymal liver. Lacerations can be classified as superficial (<3 cm in depth) or deep (>3 cm) **[19]**. Lacerations that extend to the postero superior region of segment VII may be associated with retroperitoneal hematomas around the IVC and accompanied by adrenal hematoma **[20]**. Lacerations that extend to the hepatic hilum are commonly associated with bile duct injury and are thus likely to lead to the development of a biloma. Lacerations and fractures that involve segment VI and VII follow venous path and can be extend into one or more major hepatic veins or the IVC. Such lesions are considered as major hepatic venous injuries can be life threatening and therefore are an indication for surgical treatment **[21, 22]**. When a fracture is detected, we must assess the non vascular excluded parenchyma. Large acute intraparenchymatic hematoma may be associated with perfusion trouble secondary to tissue compression and ischemia.

The detection of active contrast material extravasation at CT is important because it indicates an ongoing, potentially life-threatening hemorrhage. Several investigators clearly demonstrated that active contrast material extravasation at contrast-enhanced CT is a strong predictor of failure of nonsurgical management and recommended prompt surgical or angiographic intervention **[23-25]**.

Periportal low attenuation results as regions of low attenuation that parallel the portal vein and its branches on CT scans. Periportal low attenuation seen in proximity to a hepatic laceration may represent a hemorrhage dissecting into the periportal connective tissue. However, it can also be due to distention of the periportal lymphatic vessels secondary to elevated central venous pressure (after massive intravenous filling, high abundance pneumothorax, or pericardial tamponade **[26]**. Patients with periportal low attenuation without evidence of significant parenchymal injury can be successfully treated conservatively **[19]**.

Liver injuries are graded in severity based on CT appearance using a six-point scale **(Table 3)** according to AAST scaling that guides nonoperative management. This scaling is regarding the lesion extension and bleeding **[9]**. The AAST injury grading scale includes some criteria that cannot be assessed with CT, CT findings generally leading to underestimation of injury severity.

Liver	Injury type	Description of injury	AIS
I	Hematoma	Subscapular, <10 % surface area	2
	laceration	Capsular tear < 1 cm parenchymental depth	2
II	Hematoma	Subscapular, 10 to 50 % surface area intraparenchymaental < 10 cm in diameter	2
	laceration	Capsular tear, 1 to 3 cm parenchymental depth, < 10 cm length	2
III	Hematoma	Subscapular, > 50 % surface area of ruptured subscapular or parenchymental hematoma ;intraparenchymental hematoma> 10 cm or expending.	3
	laceration	Capsular tear > 3 cm parenchymental depth	3
IV	laceration	Parenchymal disruption involving 25 to 75 % hepatic lobe or 1 to 3 Couinaud's segments	4
V	laceration	Parenchymal disruption involving > 75 % hepatic lobe or > 3 Couinaud's segments within a single lobe	5
	vascular	Juxtahepatic venous injuries, ie, retrohepatic venacava/ central major hepatic veins	5
VI	vascular	Hepatic avulsion	6

Table 3. Alternate grading system for liver trauma [11].

Delayed CT features: delayed complications detected at follow-up CT has increased with non surgical management of liver injuries. These posttraumatic complications include delayed hemorrhage, abscess, posttraumatic pseudoaneurysm and hemobilia, and biliary complications such as biloma and bile peritonitis and are more common in patients with severe, complex liver injuries.

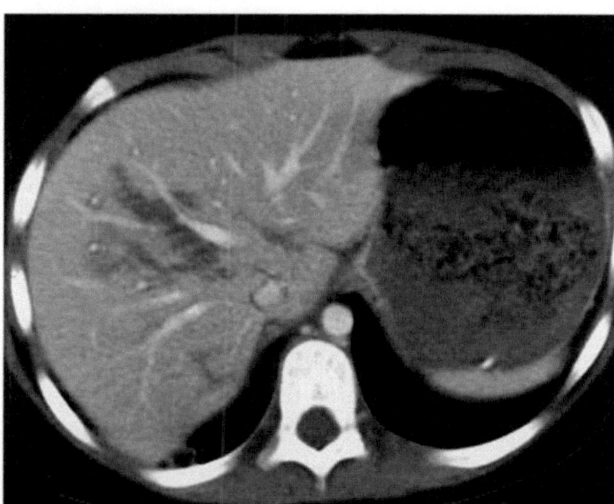

Figure 20. Multiple Lacerations of the right liver lobe that extend in the path of portal and sus-hepatic veins. These lesions are commonly associated with biliary system injury.

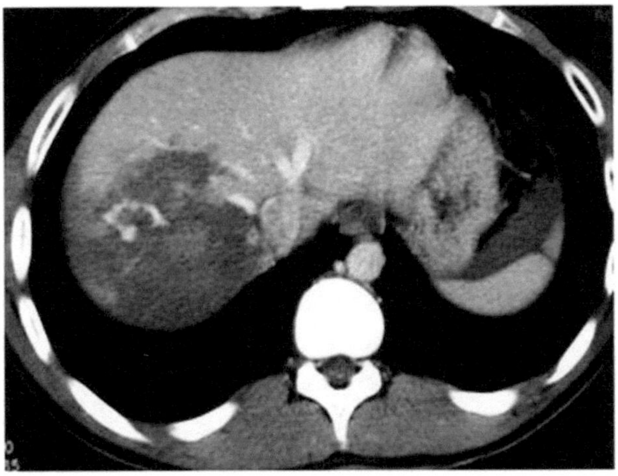

Figure 21. Grade III AAST liver injury: Contrast-enhanced CT scan shows high-attenuation foci within a hypodensity area, findings that indicate active contrast material extravasation: active bleeding.

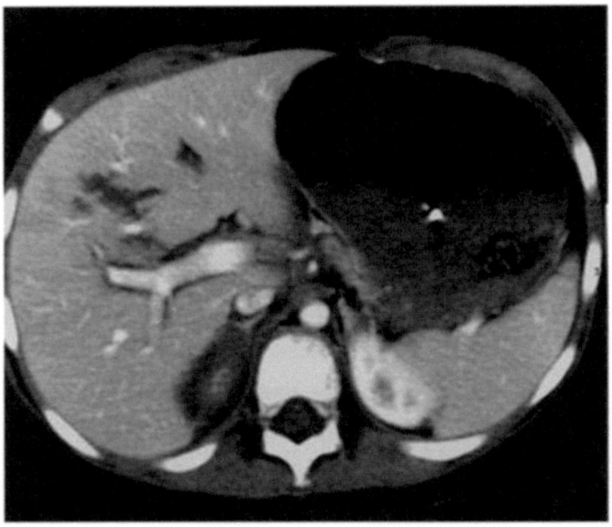

Figure 22. Periportal tracking : circumferential low attenuation areas that extend along the portal vein branches

6. Renal trauma

Urinary tract injury occurs in 10% of all abdominal trauma patients. Mechanisms of renal injuries result from Blunt renal and accounts for up to 80%–90% of all cases; Penetrating trauma accounts for approximately 10% of all renal injuries caused by gunshot or stab wounds except for the few iatrogenic injuries resulting from renal biopsy **[27]**. There is a broad consensus in favor of less invasive procedures and conservative management when a patient is stable except in cases of severe injury such as pedicle lesion or complex laceration of uretro-pelvic junction.

Contrast material–enhanced computed tomography (CT) is the imaging modality of choice in the evaluation and management of renal trauma. It can quickly and accurately depict renal injuries as well as associated injuries to other abdominal or retroperitoneal organs. It demonstrates the extent of damage tissue, perirenal hemorrhage, extravasation of urine and renal pedicle or vascular injuries. CT is important for optimal evaluation and both physiologic and morphologic information and can be obtained by using CT with contrast enhancement. The CT protocol for suspected renal trauma includes an initial arterial phase with a scanning delay of 20–30 s to identify vascular damage, followed by a nephrographic phase at 70–80 s to identify parenchymal lesions and a possible late phase at 3–20 min to detect lesions to the urinary tract **[27-30]**.

The use of MRI imaging is limited in acute renal trauma because of accessibility, motion artifacts, and the much longer scaning time than with CT.

Like for the other visceral injuries, various classification systems have been devised but the grading system of the (AAST) is widely accepted and used **(table 4) [27, 30]**.

kidney	Injury type	Description of injury	AIS
I	contusion	Microscopic or gross hematuria, urologic studies normal	2
	hematoma	Subscapsular, nonexpanding without parenchymal laceration	2
II	Hematoma	Nonexpending perirenal hematoma confirmed to renal retroperitenum	2
	laceration	< 1.0 cm parenchymal depth of renal cortex without urinary extravasation	2
III	laceration	>1.0 cm parenchymental depth of renal cortex without collecting system rupture or urinary extravasation.	3
IV	laceration	Parenchymal Laceration extending through renal cortex , medulla , and collecting system	4
	vascular	Main renal artery or vein injury with contained hemorrahge	4
V	laceration	Completely shattered kidney	5
	vascular	Avulsion of renal hilum that devascularizes kidney	5

Table 4. The American association for the surgery of trauma (AAST) renal injury severity scale **[29]**.

6.1. Grade 1 injuries

Contusions in this grade are visualized as poorly marginated round or ovoid areas of decreased enhancement and a delayed or persistent nephrogram compared with normal kidney; No evidence of contrast extravasation would be seen in the excretory phase, since the collecting system is not involved. It constitutes 75%–85% of all renal injuries in most series **[30]**. These category injuries are usually managed conservatively. A small subcapsular haematoma appears as a hypodense lesion flattening the renal capsule (**Figure 23.**). Other findings would include small subsegmental cortical infarcts (small wedge-shaped, well-defined hypodensity) and limited perinephric haematoma.

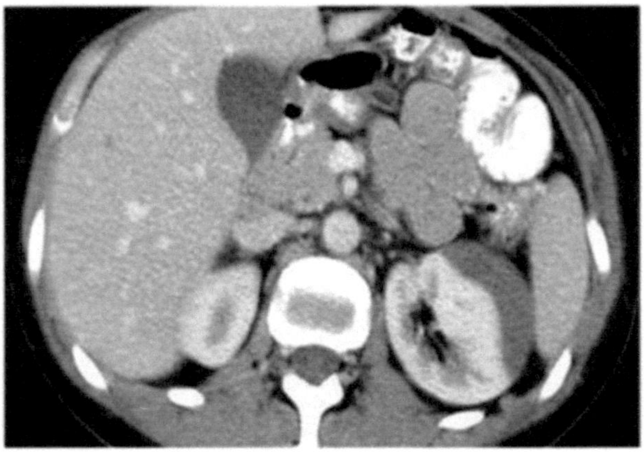

Figure 23. Axial contrast-enhanced image: Subcapsular renal hematoma with deformity of the underlying kidney (grade I AAST renal injury)

6.2. Grade II and grade III injuries

These grade include non expanding perinephric hematomas confined to the retroperitoneum and superficial cortical lacerations measuring less than 1 cm in depth (grade II) or more than 1 cm (grade III) without involvement of the collecting system (**Figure 24.**); that extend into the medulla **[29, 30]**.

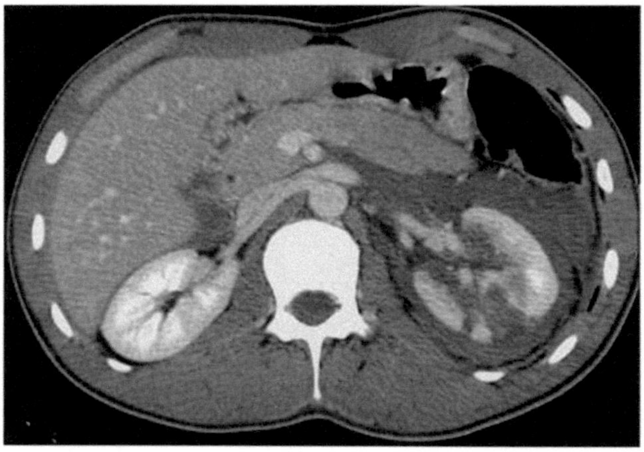

Figure 24. Axial contrast-enhanced CT scan image shows multiple lacerations of the left kidney with a mild perirenal hematoma without extension to the collecting system: grade III AAST renal injury

6.3. Grade IV injuries

Comprise cortical-medullary lacerations extending to the collecting system and injuries to the renal artery and vein with contained haemorrhage. A topographical criterion for CT recognition of injury to the calyceal system is the detection on delayed postcontrast CT images of urinary extravasion in the posterolateral perirenal space (**Figures 25., 26.**), in contrast to what happens in injuries to the renal pelvis, ureteropelvic junction or ureters, in which the urine typically collects medially at times along the course of the ureter. Urinary extravasation alone is not an indication for surgical exploration; it resolves spontaneously in approxymately 80 of cases. This grade includes segmental infarctions caused by thrombosis dissection or laceration of the segmental arteries.

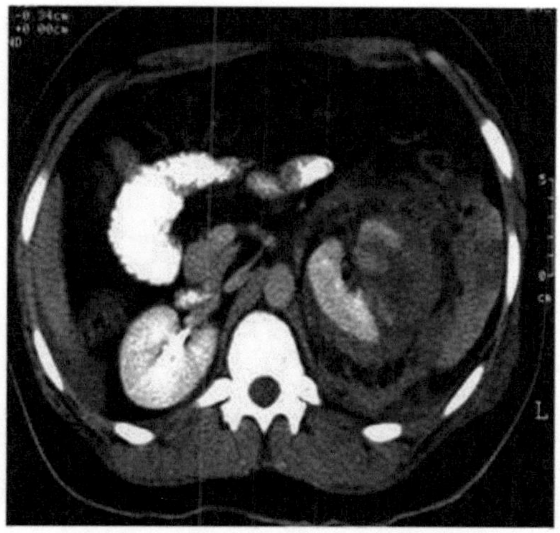

Figure 25. Axial contrast-enhanced CT scan image shows an extensive hypoperfused area of the left kidney with a large coticomedullary laceration involving collecting system. Note the perirenal haematoma.

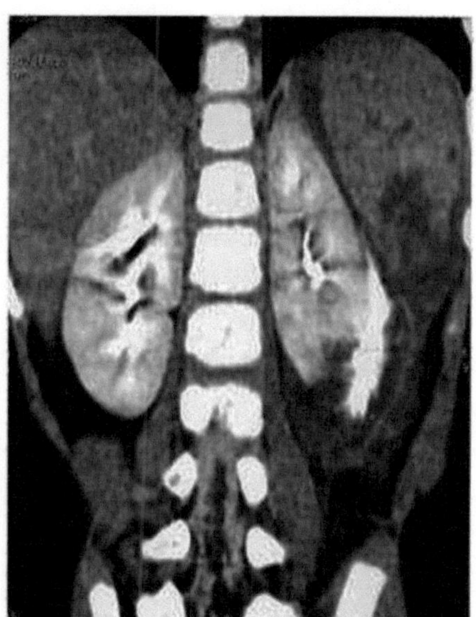

Figure 26. Delayed excretory phase CT scan with coronal reformation confirms the presence of posteroinferior urinary extravasation (arrows) (grade AAST IV renal injury)

6.4. Grade V injuries

It represent the most severe type of renal trauma and include shattered kidney which is rupture into three or more separate fragments, partial tears or complete laceration (avulsion) of the ureteropelvic junction, and thrombosis of the main renal artery or vein with devascularization of the kidney. The absence of the nephrographic effect and the presence of an extensive retroperitoneal haematoma (**Figure 27.**), especially in medial location, should raise suspicion of injury to the vascular pedicle. A typical finding is devascularisation, but more in general in arterial infarctions, is the so-called "rim sign", which is due to opacification of the capsule and subcapsular parenchyma by intact collateral capsular vessels.

Conservative management may also have a role in grade V injuries, with nephrectomy being performed in only 22% cases of major vascular trauma, in some cases deferred to 21 days after injury. It is evident that the only absolute indication for immediate exploratory surgery is the presence of "uncontrollable" active bleeding **[29, 30]**.

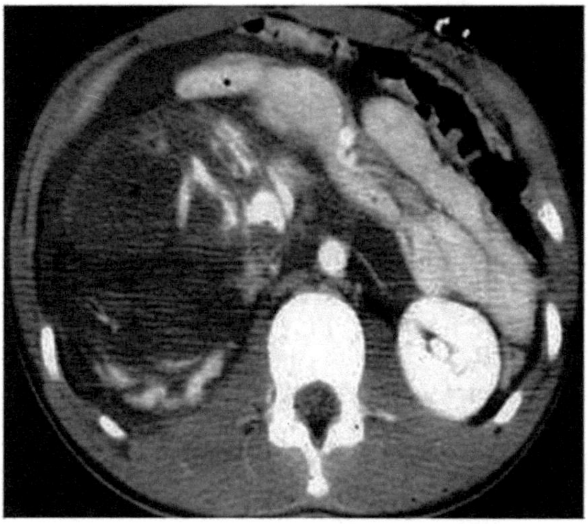

Figure 27. Axial contrast-enhanced CT scan image in venous phase: Shattered kidney with ureteropelvic junction rupture and extravasation of contrast media and avulsion of renal hilum that devascularizes the kidney (grade V AAST renal injury)

6.5. Iatrogenic renal trauma

Ultrasound-guide percutaneous core-needle biopsy is a frequently used for diagnosis of renal parenchymal disease. Biopsy complications including perirenal hematoma laceration of the renal arterial branch, arterioveinous fistula and pseudoaneurysm may occur. The majority of acquired renal arteriovenous fistulae resulting from renal biopsy heal spontaneously. Angiography can be performed effectively to achieve hemostasis.

Renal vascular injury can occur during angiography like renal artery angioplasty or a stenting procedure.Extracorporeal shock-wave litrotripsy is treatment and can lead to perirenal hematoma, (15% to 30%of cases) rupture of the kidney and lacerations **[29, 30]**.

6.6. Complications of renal trauma

Complications occur in 3% to33% of patients with renal trauma and include urinary extravasation with urinoma , infected urinoma, perinephric abcess, secondary hemorrhage secondary to a rupture of arteriovenous fistula or pseudoaneurysm.

Late or delayed complications of renal trauma develop more than 4 weeks after injury and include hypertension, hydronephrosis, calculus formation, and chronic pyelonephritis, arterioveinous fistula.

The term Page kidney refers to hypertension secondary to constrictive ischemic nephropathy caused by large chronic subcapsular hematomas, which exert a mass effect on the adjacent renal parenchyma, indenting or flattening the renal margin. **[27, 29]**.

7. Pancreatic injury

Pancreatic injuries are rare, occurring in around 2% of blunt trauma patients **[31]**, but may be associated with high morbidity and mortality, particularly if diagnosis is delayed. Indeed, the probability of complications after duodenal or pancreatic trauma ranges between 30% and 60%. Hence, early diagnosis is critical. These injuries often occur during traffic accidents as a result of the direct impact on the upper abdomen of the steering wheel or the handlebars. localisation pancreatic injuries are rarely isolated; Organ injuries most commonly associated are hepatic (46.8% of cases), gastric (42.3%), major vascular (41.3%), splenic (28.0%), renal (23.4%), and duodenal (19.3%) **[32]**.

Pancreatic injuries are often subtle and may be overlooked in patients with extensive multiorgan trauma. In 20%–40%, initial CT findings of patients with pancreatic injuries may be within normal limits in the first 12 hours after the injury **[33, 34]**. It is important to detect disruption of the pancreatic duct which is treated surgically or by therapeutic endoscopy with stent placement, while injuries without duct involvement are usually treated nonsurgically.

Today, computed tomography (CT) provides the safest and most comprehensive means of diagnosis of pancreatic injury in hemodynamically stable patients.

Serum amylase or lipase activity can be raised although in up to 40% it remains normal. Repeated testing is recommended, but results do not indicate the severity of the injury **[32]**.

7.1. CT findings in pancreatic injury

The absence of a pancreatic parenchymal phase (35–40-second delay) in whole-body CT is an obvious limitation for lesions detection. The CT findings of acute pancreatic trauma (PT) may be separated into specific (direct) features and nonspecific (indirect) features **(table5)** **[31, 35, 36]**.

Pancreas	
Direct findings	Secondary findings
Pancreatic enlargement Laceration (focal linear nonenhancement) Comminution Inhomogeneous enhancement	Peripancreatic fat stranding Peripancreatic fluid collections, which may communicate with a laceration Fluid between the splenic vein and pancreas Hemorrhage Thickening of the left anterior pararenal fascia Associated injuries to adjacent structures

Table 5. CT findings in pancreatic injuries due to blunt trauma [31].

Initial CT examination can appear normal. It is postulated that these false negative findings may result from obscuration of the fracture plane, surrounding hemorrhage, or close apposition of the pancreatic fragments **[37]**. Direct CT signs of PT include evidence of parenchymal laceration, transaction and focal enlargement or hematoma. Lacerations can be classified into superficial laceration (involving <50% of the parenchymal thickness) and deep laceration (>50% pancreatic parenchyma) (**figure 28.);** Using this cutoff can help detecting pancreatic duct disruption (**figure 29.)**. It has been shown that main duct disruption was likely present in cases of deep laceration or complete transection of the pancreatic parenchyma **[38]**. Active hemorrhage is sometimes seen. Contained vascular injuries, such as pseudoaneurysms, may also be identified on CT as evidenced by focal hyperattenuating areas which are seen to wash out on delayed phases of image acquisition **(table 6) [37].**

grade	Injury	Description
I	hematoma	Minor contusion without duct injury
	laceration	Superficial laceration without duct injury
II	Hematoma	Major contusion without duct injury
	laceration	Major laceration without duct injury
III	laceration	Distal transaction or parenchymal injury with duct injury
IV	laceration	Proximal transaction or parenchymal injury involving the ampulla or bile duct
V	disruption	Massive disruption of the pancreatique head

Table 6. Scoring pancreatic injury [31].

The indirect signs tend to be less specific when used to assess the presence of pancreatic trauma. These indirect imaging findings include peripancreatic and fat stranding and hemorrhage **[32, 39]**. Fluid between the splenic vein and the pancreas also suggests pancreatic injury. It has been shown in 90% of verified cases of blunt pancreatic trauma **[40]**. However, this finding is nonspecific.Verifying ductal status is one of the most important predictors of outcome in pancreatic trauma **[41-43]**. Any delay in diagnosis of major duct injury can result in a significant increase in mortality and direct complications such as fistula, abscess, and pseudocyst (**figure 30)**.

However, the pancreatic duct is inconsistently visualized on CT scan. New studies has shown that thinner collimation and post-processing techniques such as multiplanar reformations can improve pancreatic duct visualization **[44, 45]**.

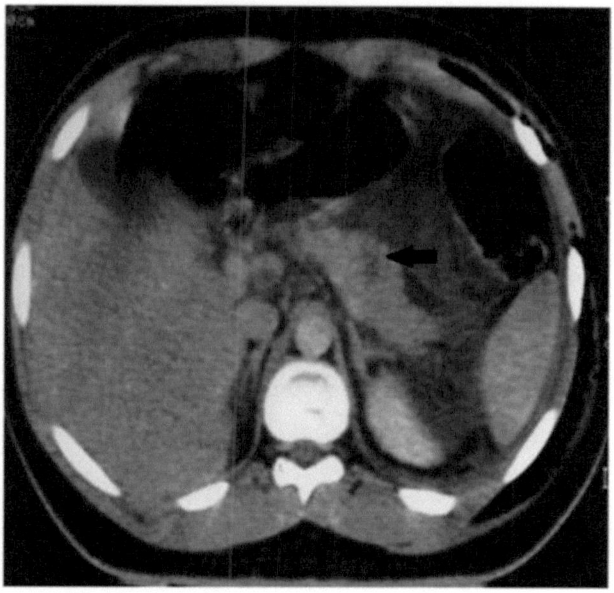

Figure 28. Contrast enhanced axial CT in the portal-venous phase demonstrates an intraparenchymal pancreatic contusion (arrow).

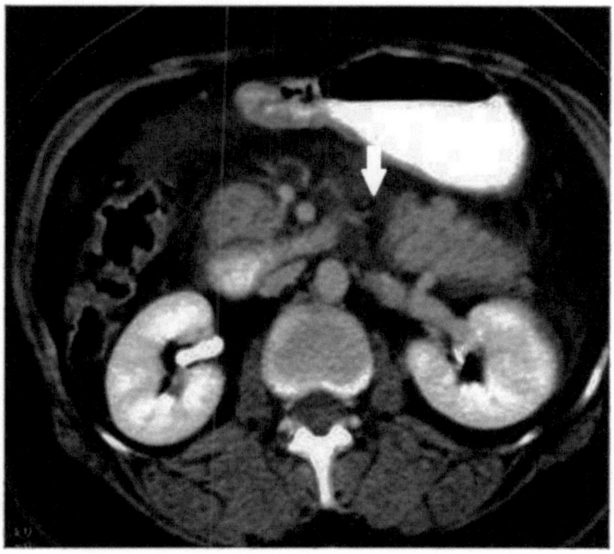

Figure 29. Contrast enhanced axial CT of a patient with a transection of the pancreas (arrow) with hemoperitoneum.

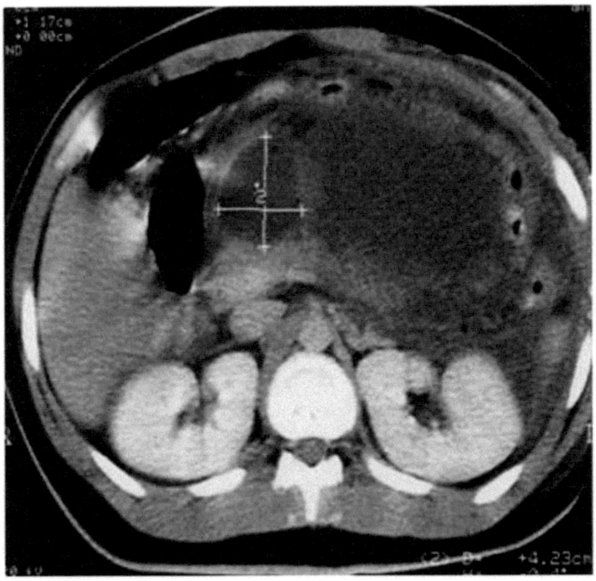

Figure 30. Large pseudocysts due to transection of the pancreatic duct several weeks after blunt

Trauma: Axial contrast-enhanced CT scan shows two large loculated fluid collections

7.2. Endoscopic Retrograde Cholangiopancreatography (ERCP)

Has been traditionally the gold standard for imaging of the pancreatic duct because of its potential to provide diagnostic images and to direct image-guided therapy. However, in the trauma setting, ERCP may not be readily available or feasible. ERCP is indicated when pancreatic injuries are detected at CT or MR imaging or if there is high clinical suspicion of ductal injury. ERCP can direct appropriate surgical repair or can be used for primary therapy by means of stent placement [31, 46].

7.3. Magnetic Resonance Cholangiopancreatography (MRCP)

Has proven a useful tool for diagnosing various abnormalities affect the pancreas and pancreatic duct. It has the ability to visualize not only the duct but also the pancreatic parenchyma and the surrounding environment **[37]**. The extension of a fracture to involve the pancreatic duct may more clearly be identified. MRI has also been found to be particularly useful in follow up of conservatively managed parenchymal injuries, fluid collections, and minor duct abnormalities **[47]**. MR follow-up plays a large role in young patients and children where minimizing cumulative radiation dose is of particular importance.

MRCP, in combination with the intravenous administration of secretin, increases pancreatic exocrine output, consequently better duct distension and delineation **[48, 49]**. Pertaining to blunt pancreatic trauma, secretin MRCP has been shown to be safe and useful in providing additional information on ductal disruption, facilitating subsequent management decisions **[49]**.

8. Biliary tract injury

Biliary tract injuries are rare following blunt trauma, occurring in only around 2% to 3% of patients undergoing laparotomy **[31]**. The most common location of biliary injury is the gallbladder, followed by the common bile duct and the intrahepatic ducts. Injuries to the gallbladder may be classified into one of three main categories: contusion, laceration/ perforation, or complete avulsion. Gallbladder injuries are difficult to recognize because of the common association to adjacent organ injury. A collapsed gallbladder or thickening (**figures 31, 32**) or disruption of the gallbladder wall suggests injury but none of these signs is specific. Pericholecystic fluid is often seen but it is not nonspecific as well.

Layering of dense fluid within the gallbladder may be an indication of intraluminal hemorrhage (**figure 33.**), although milk of calcium or excretion of intravenous contrast media from prior CT studies are pitfalls that may cause similar findings. Bile duct injury can result in free fluid, or intrahepatic bile collections **[50]**.

9. Bowel and mesenteric injuries

Are depicted in 3-5% of blunt abdominal trauma patients at laparotomy **[51-53]**, and are the third most common type of injury from blunt trauma to abdominal organs.

Delayed diagnosis of bowel and mesenteric injuries results in increased morbidity and mortality, usually because of haemorrhage or peritonitis that leads to sepsis. Three basic mechanisms may cause bowel and mesenteric injuries of blunt trauma: Direct force may crush the gastrointestinal tract; rapid deceleration may produce shearing force between fixed and mobile portions of the tract; and a sudden increase in intraluminal pressure may result in bursting injuries.

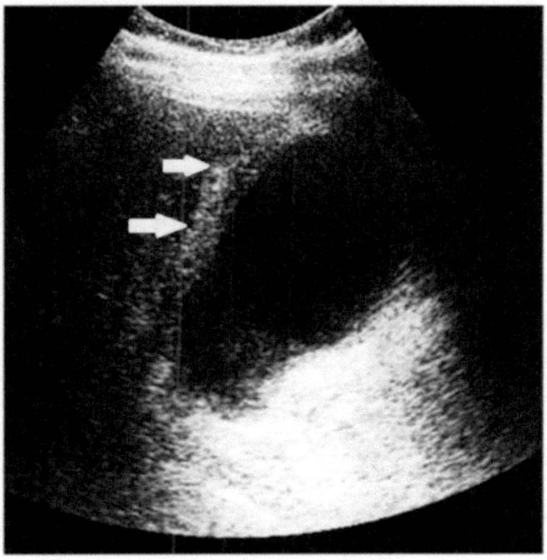

Figure 31. Post-traumatic right upper quadrant pain with fever: US shows gallbladder wall thickness (solid arrows) with intraluminal hyperechogenicities (blank arrows) mimicking cholecystitis. Surgical constatations: gallbladder avulsion, parietal necrosis, mucosal detachment (blank arrows) and peritonitis.

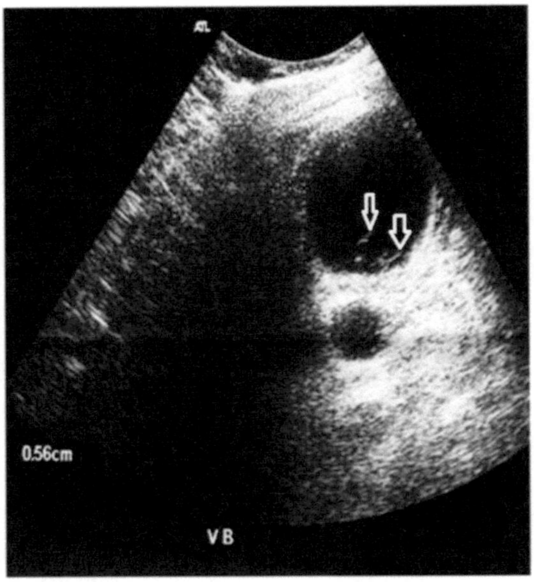

Figure 32. post-traumatic right upper quadrant pain with fever: US shows gallbladder wall thickness (solid arrows) with intraluminal hyperechogenicities (blank arrows) mimicking cholecystitis. Surgical constatations: gallbladder avulsion, parietal necrosis, mucosal detachment (blank arrows) and peritonitis.

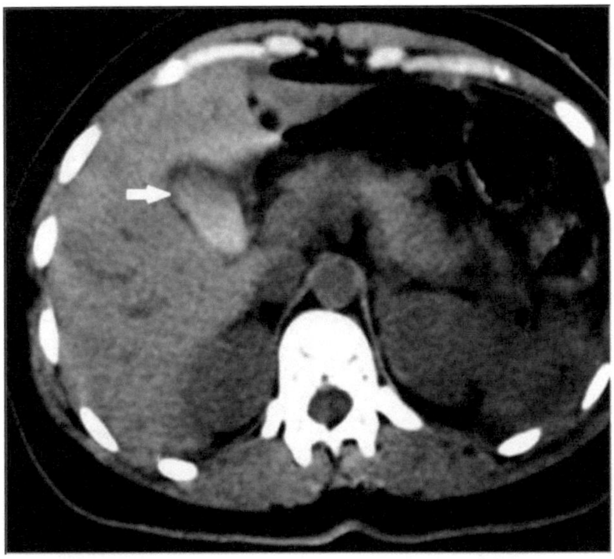

Figure 33. Dense intraluminal fluid (arrow) with collapsed gallbladder.

Multidetector CT is the most powerful tool in detecting abdominal traumatic injuries and is commonly used in evaluation of mesenteric and hollow organs lesions. It is more sensitive and specific than abdominal US.

Numerous CT signs have been described. The main goal in evaluating these signs is to distinguish significant bowel and mesenteric injuries that require surgical intervention from those that can be managed non surgically.

Helical CT scanning is very accurate in determining the need for surgical exploration in gastric injuries. However, it is less accurate in predicting the need for surgical exploration in mesenteric injuries alone

9.1. Bowel injury

Some findings are specific to bowel injury that are: bowel wall discontinuity, extraluminal contrast material and extraluminal air. Gas originating from a bowel rupture usually accumulates in locations deep to the anterior abdominal wall and may be seen also in the porta hepatis, mesentery or mesenteric veins, and portal vein.

Some patterns are not specific: bowel wall thickening, abnormal bowel wall enhancement) and mesenteric foci of fluid or fat stranding may be secondary to bowel injury alone **(Figure 34., 35.)**. Retroperitoneal air is seen with duodenal injury (**Figures 36., 37., 38.)** or the ascending or descending colon injury. Pancreatic transection should suggest duodenal injury.

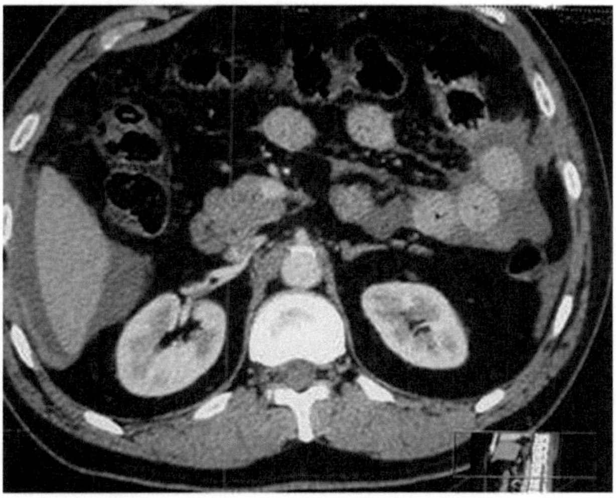

Figure 34. Traumatic perforation of jejunum : wall thickning and triangular fluid collection surrounding bowel loops

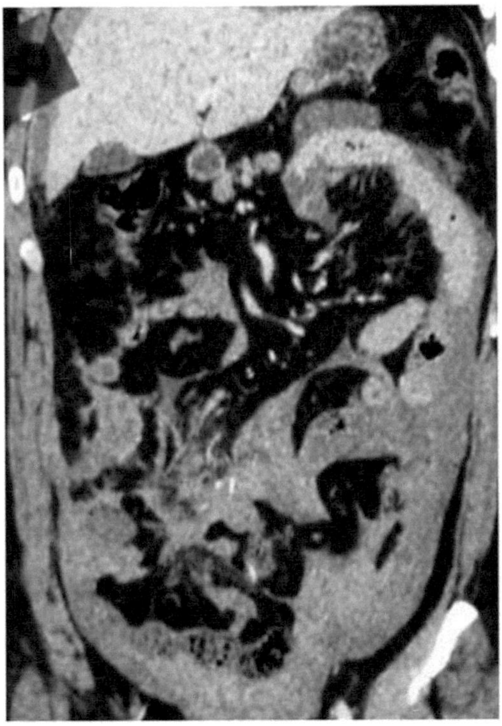

Figure 35. Traumatic perforation of jejunum : wall thickning and triangular fluid collection surrounding bowel loops

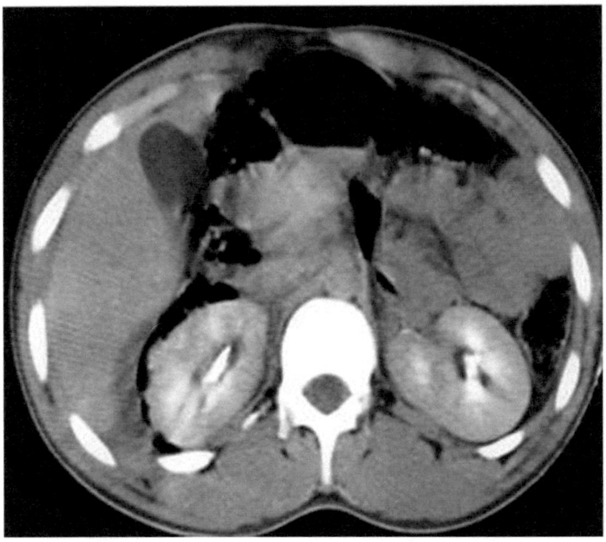

Figure 36. Iatrogenic injury of duodenum after sphincterotomy: focal retroperitoneal air surrounding the duodenum and the right perirenal space.

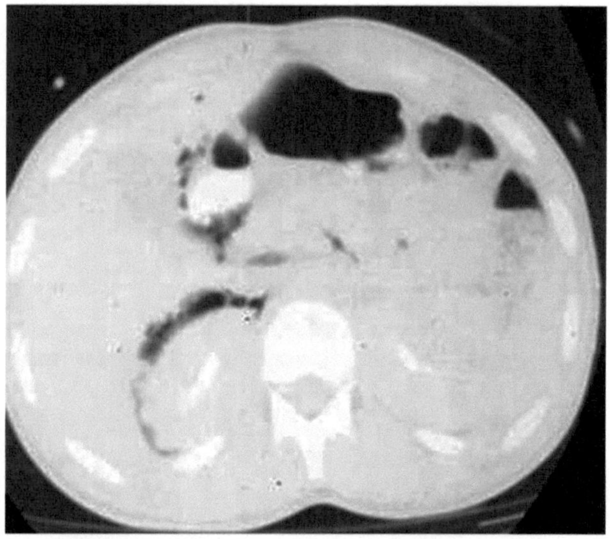

Figure 37. Same patient and same axial CT scan on lung window: free retroperitoneal air revealed as foci of low attenuation

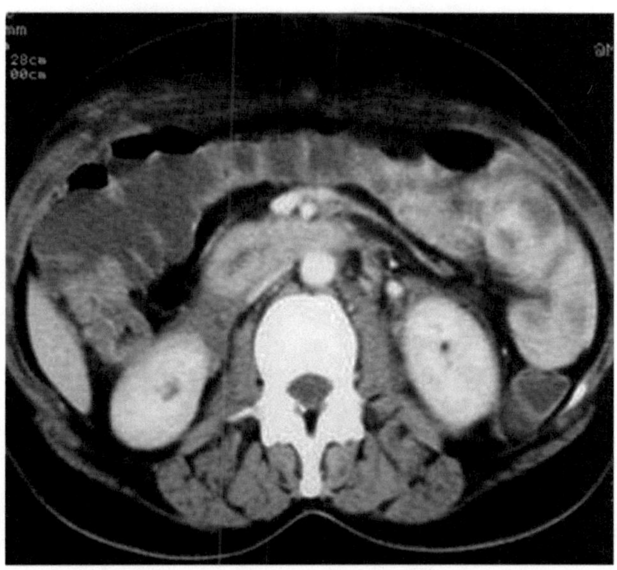

Figure 38. Intramural hematoma of duodenum ; circumferential thickening and intense enhancement of the wall.

9.2. Isolated mesenteric injuries

Significant mesenteric injuries include active mesenteric bleeding, disruption of the mesentery, and mesenteric injury associated with bowel ischemia. An isolated mesenteric hematoma is considered non significant **[51, 54]**.

Acute bleeding may occur from the small mesenteric vessels, and signs of intra-peritoneal blood loss make early laparotomy imperative. Injuries to the main mesenteric vessels resulting in acute haemorrhage are rare; Bowel infarction may result from either mesenteric tears with disruption of blood vessels or mesenteric vessel thrombosis, either venous or arterial: Mesenteric extravasation. This sign has a specificity of 100% for the diagnosis of significant mesenteric injury, but it was seen in only nine (17%) of 54 patients with bowel and mesenteric injuries inding of mesenteric extravasation is usually an indication for urgent lap **(Figure 39., 40., 41.)**.

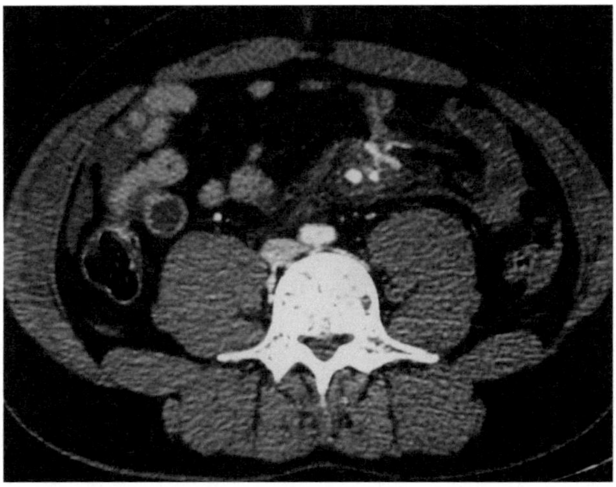

Figure 39. Bowel and Mesenteric injury : mesenteric contrast extravasation, vascular beading and fat stranding

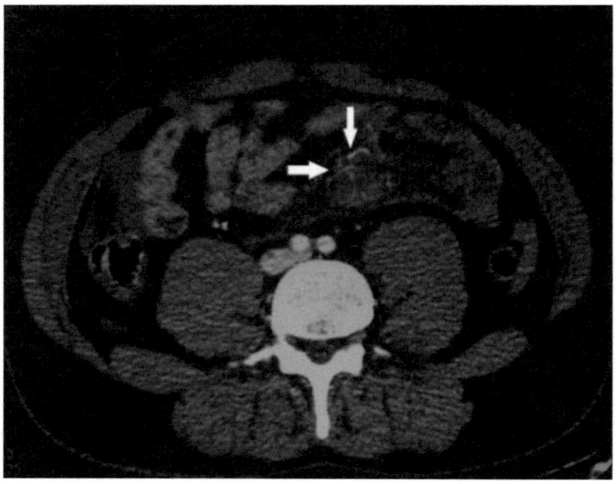

Figure 40. Bowel and Mesenteric injury : mesenteric contrast extravasation, vascular beading and fat stranding

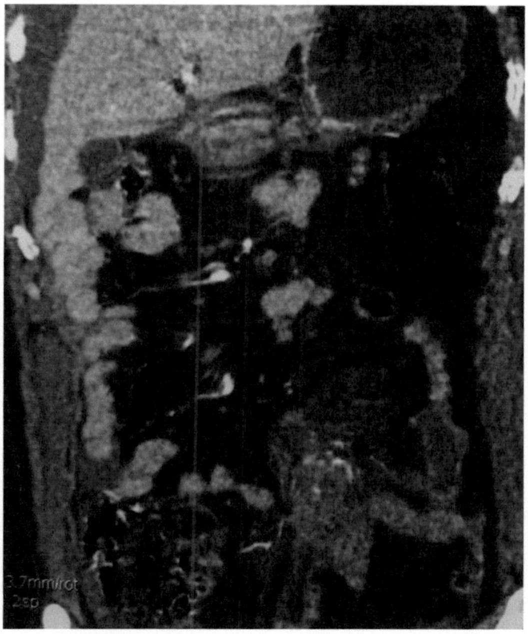

Figure 41. Bowel and Mesenteric injury : mesenteric contrast extravasation, vascular beading and fat stranding

9.2.1. Mesenteric vascular beading

This feature appears on CT images as an irregularity in mesenteric vessels; like mesenteric extravasation of contrast material, it is indicative of vascular injury.

Termination of mesenteric vessels. Abrupt termination of a mesenteric artery or vein is also an indication of vascular injury.

Less specific findings as Mesenteric infiltration may indicate mesenteric injury with or without bowel wall injury. Mesenteric Hematoma seen as a well-defined mesenteric hematoma indicative of laceration of a mesenteric vessel **[54]**.

10. Colonic injury

Compression of the upper abdomen caused by a steering wheel or lap-type seat belts appears to predispose patients to colonic injury.

The transverse colon, sigmoid and caecum portions are the most common sites of injury.

CT findings are intramural hematoma especially on the transverse colon, avulsion of the mesentery, full thicknes- laceration, transaction and devascularisation are seen in injuries of ascendin and descending colon **[55]**.

11. Gastric traumatic injuries

Are rare, secondary to penetrating or blunt trauma. The incidence of blunt gastric trauma is estimated between 0.4% and 1.7% of all abdominal traumas **[51, 52]**.

Blunt trauma lesions are more often the consequence of a high velocity impact involving the epigastric region in post-meal phase, since an important condition to occur is gastric fullness **[53, 54]**. Trauma may produce a gastric rupture, more frequently observed at the fundus (**figures 42, 43, 44**).

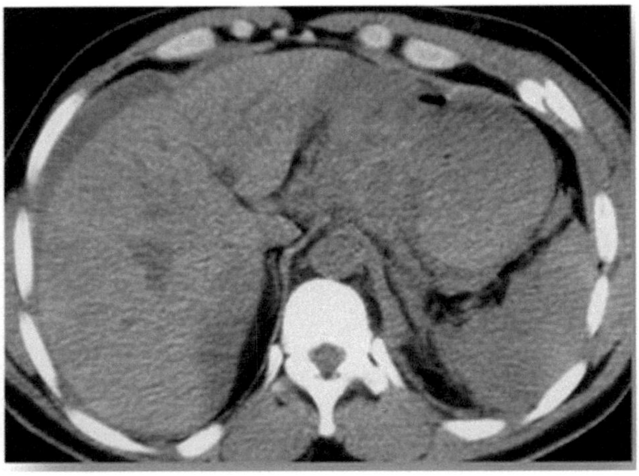

Figure 42. Fundus rupture with antral wall contusion that appears spontaneously hyperdense, Large volume of intraperitoneal fluid with active bleeding, extraluminal air (pneumoperitoneum), spleen complete shuttering and liver contusion

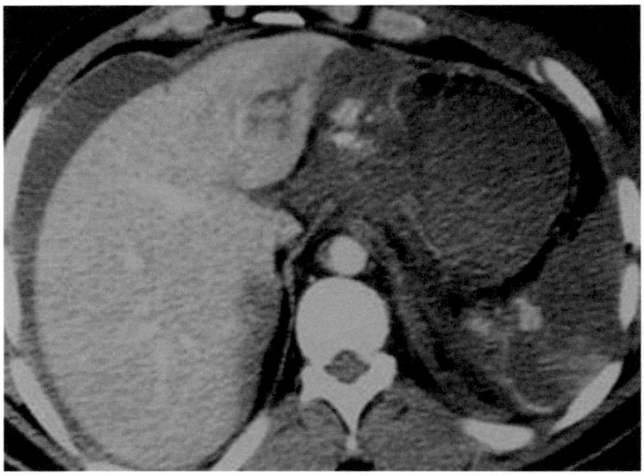

Figure 43. Fundus rupture with antral wall contusion that appears spontaneously hyperdense, Large volume of intraperitoneal fluid with active bleeding, extraluminal air (pneumoperitoneum), spleen complete shuttering and liver contusion

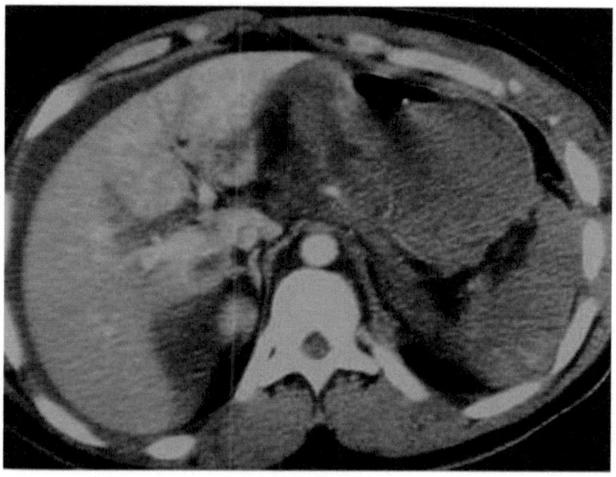

Figure 44. Fundus rupture with antral wall contusion that appears spontaneously hyperdense, Large volume of intraperitoneal fluid with active bleeding, extraluminal air (pneumoperitoneum), spleen complete shuttering and liver contusion

As in traumatic injuries of other abdominal organs, peritoneal fluid indicates a relevant lesion, mainly if it is bloody. The gas content of the stomach usually plays a protective role; sometimes it can dissect the mucosal layer and pass into the gastric veins. In these cases, portal pneumatosis may happen **[56]**. It is important to be aware of this condition because it is possible to misinterpret the pneumatosis as a consequence of an intestinal infarction due to the traumatic shock. It is also very important to play attention to gas considered that pneumoperitoneum is observed in almost all patients having a complete gastric rupture **[50]**.

CT findings in intestinal perforation can be subtle and nonspecific. Wall thickening, wall discontinuity, extraluminal air, and mesenteric hematoma **(figures 45, 46)** are reasonably specific CT signs. The presence of a moderate to large volume of intraperitoneal fluid without visible solid organ injury is an important sign.

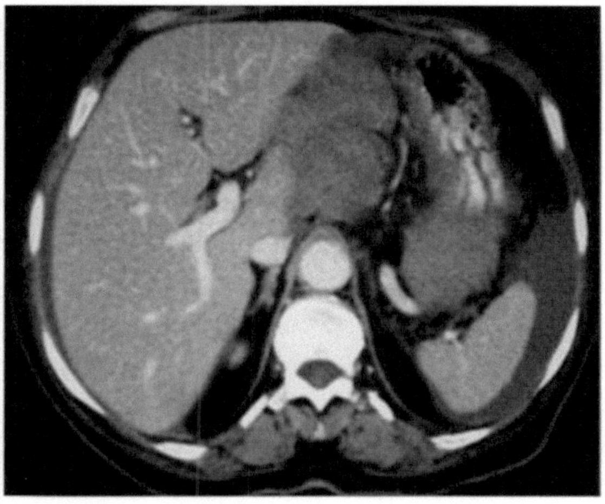

Figure 45. Contrast-enhanced CT scan with contrast ingestion: Posterior wall gastric hematoma, epiploic hematoma and intraperitoneal fluid

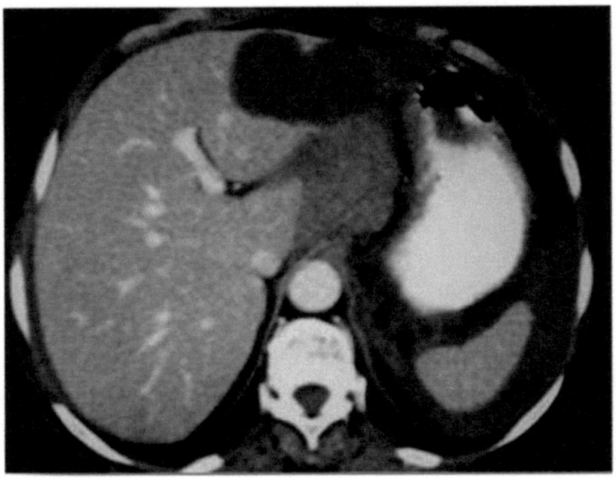

Figure 46. Contrast-enhanced CT scan with contrast ingestion: Posterior wall gastric hematoma, epiploic hematoma and intraperitoneal fluid

12. Diaphragmatic injury

The diaphragm may be injured by penetrating or blunt trauma. Diaphragmatic breach without visceral injury or herniation may be difficult to detect due to a paucity of clinical signs and herniation may be misdiagnosed following the wrong interpretation of chest radiology. If not recognized there is a considerable risk of late morbidity and mortality.

Plain chest radiography is the first technique to prefer. When performed immediately after the accident, it presents a suspicion about the diagnosis of a ruptured diaphragm in only 20–34% of the cases **[57-59]**. Diaphragmatic injury is shown as a soft-tissue opacity, containing visceral gas in the thorax, which is pathognomonic of diaphragmatic hernia). It also reveals associated rib fractures and haemopneumothorax. Although the strangulated bowel presents as intrathoracic air-fluid levels, the perforated bowel presents as pneumothorax. If there is a bowel obstruction, plain radiography of the abdomen shows air-fluid levels with abdominal distension **[60]**. The detection of a nasogastric tube above the left hemidiaphragm is a possible imaging feature.

CT examination of abdomen and thorax is a very useful and reliable tool in the evaluation of diaphragmatic injury. Multiplanar reformations are expected to improve sensitivity. CT can demonstrate findings consistent with diaphragmatic injury, such as diaphragmatic discontinuity, thickened diaphragm signs, intrathoracic herniation of abdominal contents, and waist-like constriction of abdominal viscera (the 'collar sign') **[60-62]**, **(Figures 47., 48.)**. An abnormal hepatic location depicted on axial CT can be considered as a potentially indirect sign of right diaphragm rupture with liver herniation. The so-called "dependent viscera" sign (when the upper one third of the liver abuts the posterior right ribs or whether the bowel or stomach lays in contact with the posterior left ribs) is nearly 100% specific **[63]**. The diaphragm itself may be obscured by hemothorax or hemoperitoneum.

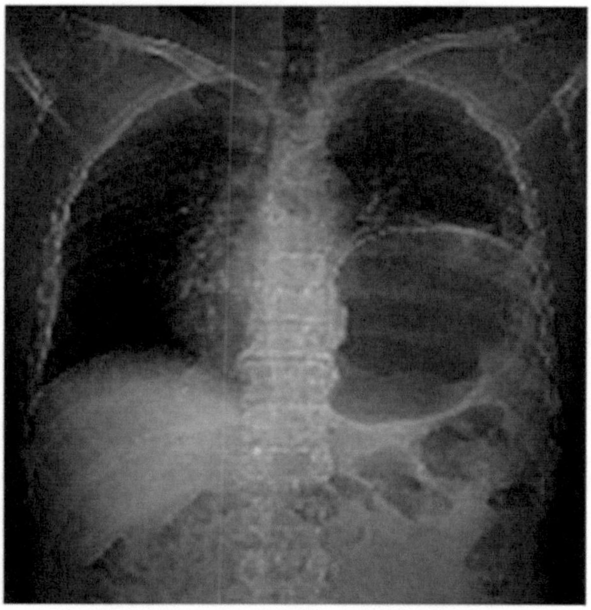

Figure 47. 42 years-old man with post-traumatic acute epigastragia, dysphagia and deshydration. Scout-view CT scan showing left intrathoracic visceral gas. Sagittal reformatted image confirm diaphragmatic hernia of the stomach with the collar sign and intra-thoracic fluid-air level.

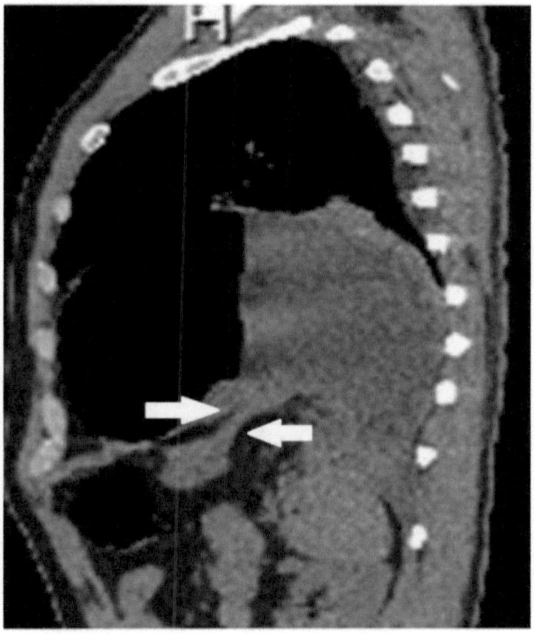

Figure 48. 42 years-old man with post-traumatic acute epigastragia, dysphagia and deshydration. Scout-view CT scan showing left intrathoracic visceral gas. Sagittal reformatted image confirm diaphragmatic hernia of the stomach with the collar sign and intra-thoracic fluid-air level.

13. Pelvic trauma

13.1. Arterial bleeding in pelvic trauma

Vascular injuries are a major source of morbidity and mortality in patients with blunt pelvic trauma. Bleeding is usually of venous origin. However, in 10%-20% of the patients, hemodynamic instability is associated with arterial hemorrhage. Mortality of up to 50% has been reported despite effective control of bleeding.

Pelvic CT angiography is useful in assessing vascular injuries and provides a complete study of bone, visceral and especially vascular lesions. Contrast-enhanced CT has been reported to be an accurate, noninvasive technique for identifying ongoing arterial hemorrhage in patients with pelvic fractures **[64-68]**.

MDCT angiography study technique is able to identify the presence of active bleeding with the possibility in some cases of defining the source of the blood loss with a sensitivity of 66%– 90%, a specificity of 85%–98%, and an accuracy of 87%–98% being reported **[66-67, 69-70]**. High-quality multiplanar reconstructions provide a reliable vascular map of the anatomical structures **(Figures 49., 50.)**. This technique is highly predictive of arterial injury that will require angiographic embolization **[67], (Figures 51., 52.)**. The most important differential diagnosis is the clotted blood from which it is distinguished by measuring CT attenuation. Active bleeding shows higher attenuation.

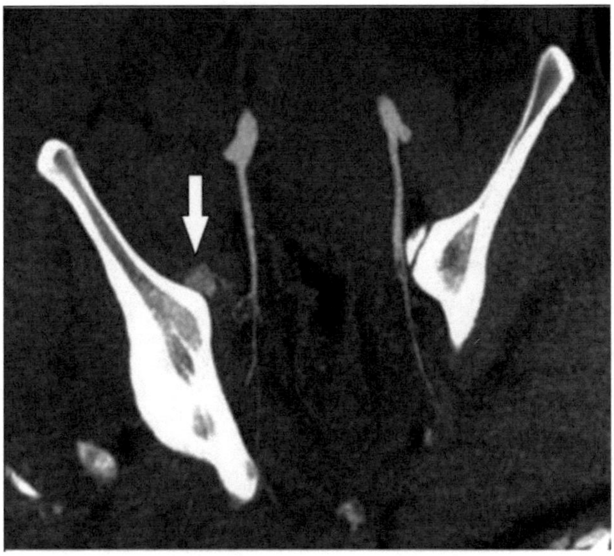

Figure 49. CT-angiographic correlation for detection of bleeding from a branch of the internal iliac artery. Contrast-enhanced CT scan in an arterial phase with coronal oblique reformation

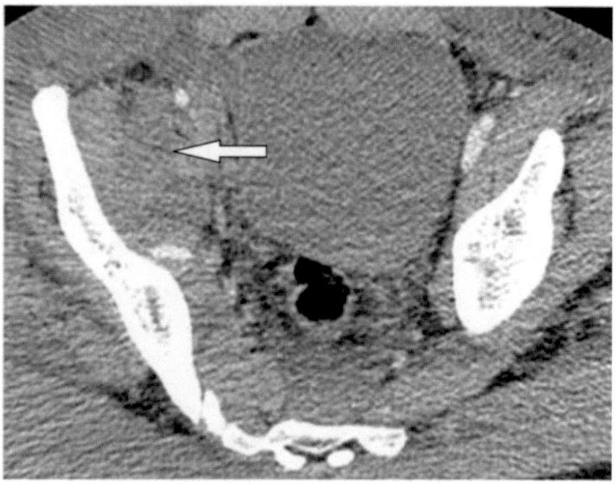

Figure 50. CT-angiographic correlation for detection of bleeding from a branch of the internal iliac artery. Axial image after contrast-enhanced CT scan in a portal-venous phase: extravasation of contrast material within a hematoma of the right iliacus muscle.

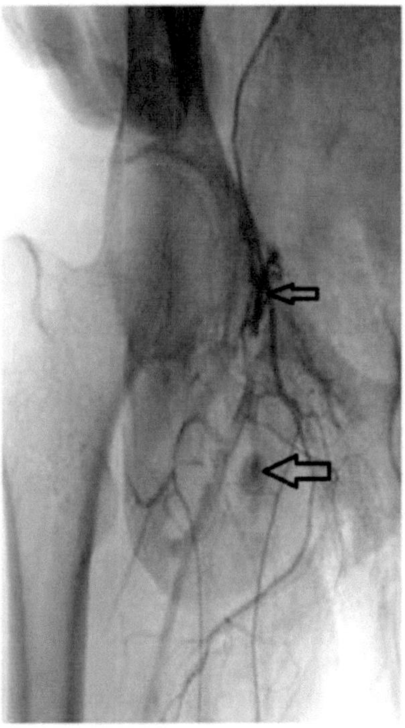

Figure 51. CT-angiographic correlation for detection of bleeding from a branch of the internal iliac artery. Angiogram shows multifocal extravasation (arrows) of branches of right internal artery.

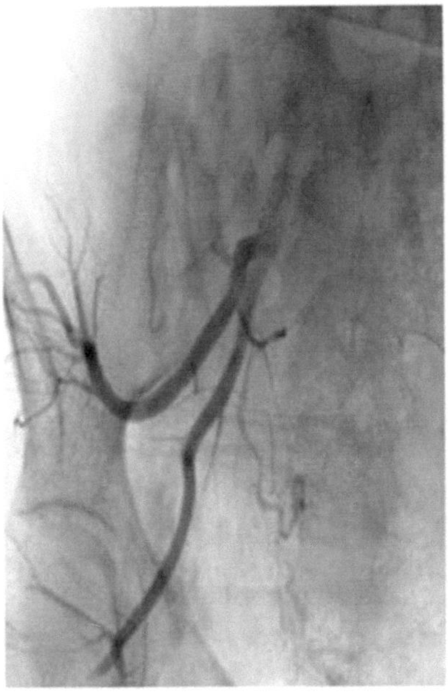

Figure 52. CT-angiographic correlation for detection of bleeding from a branch of the internal iliac artery. Right internal iliac arteriogram obtained after embolization shows no further hemorrhage.

In patients with pelvic trauma, the arterial vessels most frequently injured are the branches of the internal iliac artery, whereas the external iliac artery is less frequently involved.

The detection of contrast material extravasation on CT scans facilitates urgent angiography and subsequent transcatheter embolisation which are the most effective methods for controlling ongoing arterial bleeding and can be life-saving **[71]**.

14. Place of interventional radiology in the management of trauma abdominals

Hemostasis and revascularization. Hemorrhagic lesions can be divided into visceral and vascular injuries pure. They may benefit from percutaneous embolization techniques, Dissections and traumatic thrombosis benefit from percutaneous revascularization due to recent technical advances **[72]**.

14.1. Interventional radiology of hemostasis

14.1.1. Principles and technique

14.1.1.1. General principles

When the diagnosis of traumatic hemorrhagic parenchymal lesion and / or vascular was posed hemostasis is obtained by percutaneous embolization via a catheter angiography The technique is significantly different of embolization techniques for tumor or arteriovenous malformation by answering threecrucial points:

- The temporary embolization using absorbable material is usually sufficient to generate the local formation of thrombus. The recanalization of the occluded vessel secondary is not a problem.
- Vascular occlusion must always be performed at the site colitis.
- Embolization does not cause tissue damage, or at least minimally.

14.1.1.2. Vascular access

The percutaneous access is usually right or left femur. The use of bony landmarks under fluoroscopy or ultrasound guidance are quickly implemented in case of difficulty puncture order not to waste time on vascular access. If the patient already has an arterial access we can "take" it as an access. The use of a vascular introducer (désilet) 5-French is very useful to allow the rapid exchange catheter. In large pelvic trauma or major skin and muscle deformities, a brachial access is necessary **[72-73]**.

14.1.1.3. Catheterization

If the patient has already received a CT scan with injection of iodinated contrastThe catheterization will be immediately on known or suspected bleeding sites. Without scanner, the aortography face must be systematic to guide the selective catheterization. negativity of aortography does not rule out the presence of hemorrhagic lesions that only selective series can deny. The most commonly used catheters are pre-formed type Cobra and Simmons. Caliber 4 or 5-French, they can usually make the diagnosis and treatment. In case of difficult catheterization or to embolize very selectively, Recent advances in materials make available micro-catheter 2 or 3-French highly efficient and capable of delivering micro-emboli **[72-73]**.

14.1.1.4. Emboli and embolization

The Curaspon®, temporary embolus type animal gelatin which disappears within three weeks the best embolus Fragments of variable size and shape are used according to the habits of each; Only the use of this product powder is clearly inadvisable. Indeed, as the particles PVA (polyvinyl alcohol), who also have the drawback of being definitive emboli, powder provides a very distal embolization, which has no interest in this context and can generate extensive visceral infarcts and abscesses. The coils, final emboli formed by coiling optionally covered with thrombogenic fibers, are widely used in certain territories or failure of Curaspon® may occur in case of major disruption of hemostasis. The use of biological glue Histo-Acryl ®-type (n-butylcyanoacrylate) which polymerizes in contact with basic environments such as water or blood is possible in case of difficulties in obtaining satisfactory embolization with other emboli. It should not be used in first intention. Final bolus, its handling requires great skill and its use in the context of trauma that is the subject of rare publications.

14.1.2. Embolization of visceral injuries

Most teams currently recognize conservative nonsurgical treatment as the standard treatment of hemodynamically stable patients the exploration and surgical treatment remain the reference of unstable patients. It is within this context of conservative treatment that is positioned interventional radiology, the indications are in many assessment teams without well-defined consensual attitude to this day.

14.1.2.1. Splenic injury

Conservative treatment, strict bed rest and Surveillance, is supposed to be the reference, we are surprised by a great heterogeneity of findings with failure rates between 2 and 52%. Moreover, some studies have shown that a hemoperitoneum greater than 300 ml, a high grade lesion scannographic and / or the presence of a leak active contrast or a« blush » scanner to be risk factors for failure. These patients would thus theoretically good candidates for further treatment by embolization. Once the indication for embolization posed, remains the choice of technique, currently being discussed in the literature: selective embolization of vascular lesions viewed or proximal embolization of the splenic artery trunk by coils. The first one, theoretically longer would be associated with more frequent and extensive splenic infarction. The second concept is to reduce the intra-splenic pression to allow hemostasis while leaving the possibility of a resumption of the splenic blood supply by the short gastric vessels. The addition of embolization achieves failure rates below 10% among patients with high-grade lesions. Remains the poorly known problem of residual splenic function after embolization **[74-76]**.

14.1.2.2. Liver injury

As for the spleen, indications of hepatic arterial chemoembolization remain to be defined. Both indications are currently the most common: the persistent déglobulisation in a traumatized liver and the detection of contrast leakage or intraparenchymal blush on CT. Embolization should be here as selective as possible. The series of the literature report success rates of 90-100% and low morbidity **[74, 77, 78]**.

14.1.2.3. Kidney injury

The arteriovenous embolization was reported in cases of extravasation of contrast, of arteriovenous fistula or pseudoaneurysm with a very high efficiency. The embolization should be as selective as possible to preserve as much renal parenchyma as possible, most often using microcatheters and microcoils. In the extended or proximal forms, the embolization of renal artery trunk is possible, To control bleeding and avoid nephrectomy of hemostasis, act often dreaded by surgeons **[79-80]**.

14.1.3. Vascular injuries "pure"

14.1.3.1. Pelvic injuries

Conducted immediately in a patient carrying an unstable pelvic fracture or secondarily after visualization of a pelvic active leak, the embolization of internal iliac territories will be selective if possible **(Figure 51., 52.)**

The involved branches are in decreasing order of frequency: superior gluteal, lateral sacral, iliolumbar, obturator, inferior gluteal .The selective catheterization, however, can be long. And the proximal internal iliac embolization unilateral or bilateral must be the first option in the very unstable patients. Conventionally carried out using Curaspon ®, the embolization may be supplemented with coils in case of bleeding disorders after massive transfusion. The internal iliac embolization is now a mature technology, efficient (90-100% control of bleeding) and safe **[72, 81]**.

14.1.3.2. Retroperitoneal injuries

The lumbar and iliolumbar arteries are most often involved. The Bleeding may also come from other arteries: intercostal, inferior phrenic, adrenal, pancreaticoduodenal. Two elements are crucial when we are led to embolize thoracolumbar territories:

- The origin of the anterior spinal artery must be tracked and the embolization carried out downstream thereof where appropriate.
- The levels metameric arteries above and underlies a lumbar artery should be embolized to prevent further bleeding by the physiological interlombaires anastomoses **[72, 81]**.

14.2. Interventional radiology of revascularization

The introduction of stents has been described as in traumatic dissections of the renal artery in clinical cases or small series. This is made possible by the knowledge and technical developments derived from acquired coronary stenting. The period of treatment remains unclear: the theoretical threshold of 6 hours of ischemia could be the rule but recent work has shown the absence of renal functional benefit for revascularization (endovascular or surgical) beyond 4 hours of warm ischemia.

15. Conclusion

Beyond the diagnosis, the radiologist offers, through technological advances, of minimally invasive treatment options, fast, available, efficient and more mature. Thus, progress of interventional radiology in trauma residing longer in the indications progress that in the techniques progress between the "all surgical" and "all conservative", the various interventional techniques have certainly an important place to take.

16. Gunshot wounds

Surgical exploration of abdominal gunshot wound victims has been the standard of care for the greater part of the last century, The accumulating evidence demonstrate, however, that taking all abdominal gunshot wound victims to laparotomy leads to a negative or non-therapeutic procedure in 15% to 25% of cases **[82-85]**.

The management of hemodynamically stable abdominal gunshot wound victims has been changing in the last few years and has been gradually replaced by a conservative strategy. Diagnostic imaging methods are providing information which could help with a more appropriate treatment decision. Abdominal plain radiographies are used to search for pneumoperitoneum and to identify the location and number of retained projectiles. Ultrasonography is less used in penetrating trauma. The role of CT in evaluating hemodynamically stable blunt abdominal trauma patients is well established, and CT became the imaging modality of choice in this situation **[36]**. Lesions may involve solid and/or hollow organs, the urinary bladder, vessels, diaphragm and bones. MDCT is safely used to determine projectile trajectory and likely injuries **(figure 53., 54., 55)**.

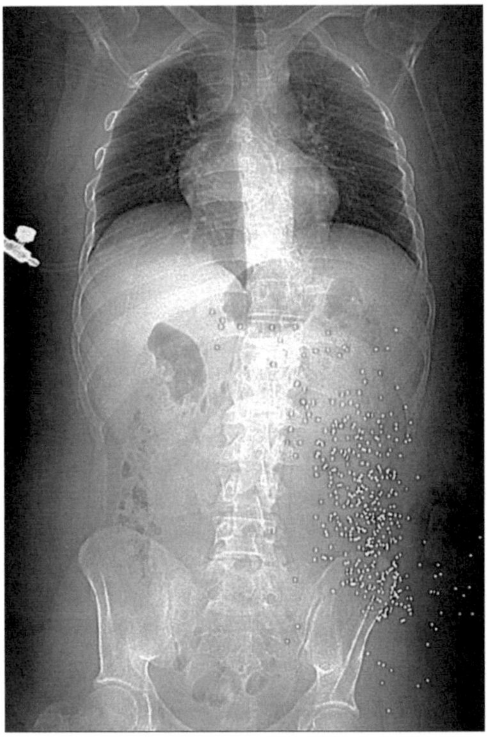

Figure 53. Penetrating abdominal injury. Chest and abdominal x-ray (scout view) shows the location and the profusion of retained projectiles.

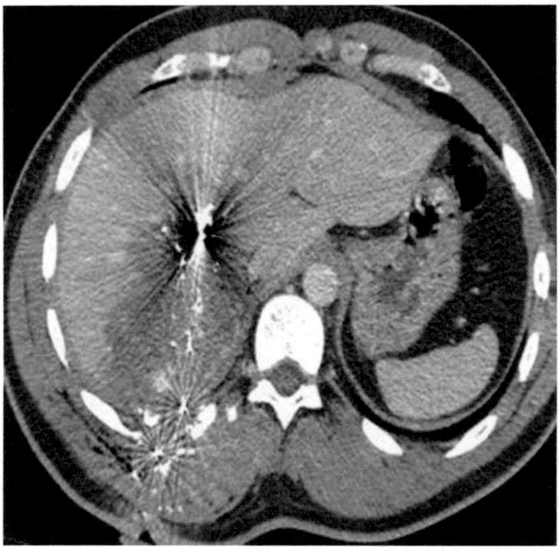

Figure 54. Penetrating abdominal injury. CT with IV contrast (soft-tissue window) shows a large hypodense area indicating hepatic contusion.

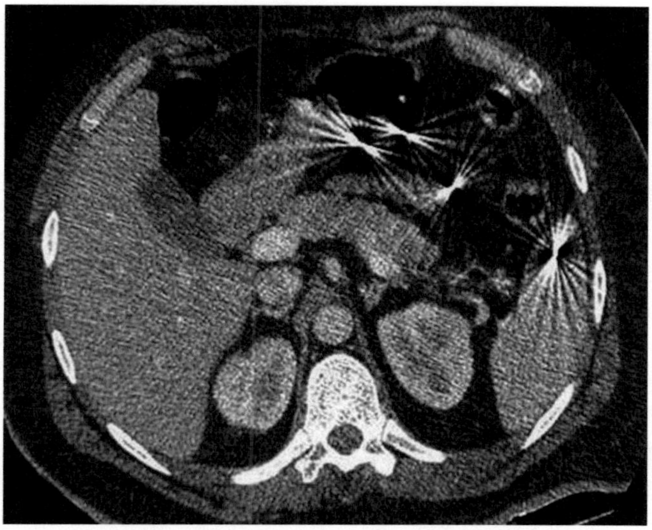

Figure 55. Penetrating abdominal injury. Shows intra-abdominal location of retained projectiles.

17. Conclusion

Abdominal trauma represents an important part of daycare activity in radiology. Nonsurgical treatment has become the standard of care in hemodynamically stable patients with abdominal trauma as a result of exhaustive and rigorous assessment of injury lesions by imaging. US is a non invasive readily available method of detection of free fluid in trauma patient; the fast exam looks for intraperitoneal and intrapericardial anechoic fluid and allows selection of patients for CT. CT is the technique of choice for initial examination of hemodynamically stable patients after abdominal trauma because it is highly sensitive, specific and accurate in detecting the presence or absence of injury and defining its extend.

Author details

Nadia Mama*, Hela Jemni, Nadia Arifa Achour, Ould Chavey Sidiya,
Kaled Kadri, Mehdi Gaha, Ibtisem Hasni and Kalthoum Tlili
Department of Radiology, Sahloul Hospital, Sousse, Tunisia

18. References

[1] Ultrasonography for the diagnosis of intraperitoneal free air in chest-abdominal-pelvic blunt trauma and critical acute abdominal pain. Arch Surg. 2009; 144(2):137-41.

[2] Cokkinos D, Antypa E, Stefanidis K, Tserotas P, Kostaras V, Parlament A, Tavernaraki K, Piperopoulos PN. Contrast-enhanced ultrasound for imaging blunt abdominal trauma - indications, description of the technique and imaging review. Ultraschall Med. 2012; 33(1): 60-7.

* Corresponding Author

[3] Branney SW, Wolfe RE, Moore EE. et *al.* Quantitative sensitivity of ultrasound in detecting free intraperitoneal fluid. J Trauma. 1995; 39: 375–380.

[4] Goodman CS, Hur JY, Adajar MA et *al.* How well does CT predict the need for laparotomy in hemodynamically stable patients with penetrating abdominal injury? A review and meta-analysis. AJR Am J Roentgenol. 2009; 193: 432–437.

[5] Shanmuganathan K, Mirvis SE, Boyd-Kranis R et al. Nonsurgical management of blunt splenic injury: use of CT criteria to select patients for splenic arteriography and potential endovascular therapy. Radiology. 2000; 217: 75–82.

[6] Shanmuganathan K, Mirvis SE, Sherbourn CD, et al. Hemoperitoneum as the sole indicator of abdominal visceral injuries: a potential limitation of screening abdominal US for trauma. Radiology. 1999; 212(2) :423-430.

[7] Wing VW, Federle MP, Morris JA Jr, et al. The clinical impact of CT for blunt trauma. AJR Am J Roentgenol. 1985; 145: 1191-1194.

[8] Clark TJ, Cardoza S, Kanth N. Splenic trauma: pictorial review of contrast-enhanced CT findings. Emerg Radiol. 2011; 18(3): 227-34.

[9] Moore EE, Shackford SR, Pachter HL, McAninch JW, Browner BD, Champion HR, Flint LM, Gennarelli TA, Malangoni MA, Ramenofsky ML, et al. Organ injury scaling: spleen, liver, and kidney. J Trauma. 1989; 29(12): 1664-6.

[10] Tinkoff G, Esposito TJ, Reed J, Kilgo P, Fildes J, Pasquale M, Meredith JW. American Association for the Surgery of Trauma Organ Injury Scale I: spleen, liver, and kidney, validation based on the National Trauma Data Bank. J Am Coll Surg. 2008 ;207(5):646-55.

[11] Marmery H, Shanmuganathan K, Alexander M et al. Optimization of selection for nonoperative management of blunt splenic injury: comparison of MDCT grading systems. AJR. 2007; 189: 1421–1427.

[12] Matthes G, Stengel D, Seifert J, et al. Blunt liver injuries in polytrauma: results from a cohort study with the regular use of whole-body helical computed tomography. World J Surg. 2003; 27:1124–1130.

[13] Romano L, Giovine S, Guidi G, Tortora G, Cinque T, Romano S. Hepatic trauma: CT findings and considerations based on our experience in emergency diagnostic imaging. Eur J Radiol. 2004; 50(1):59-66.

[14] Croce MA, Fabian TC, Menke PG, et al. Nonoperative management of blunt hepatic trauma is the treatment of choice for hemodynamically stable patients: results of a prospective trial. Ann Surg. 1995; 221:744–755

[15] Pachter HL, Spencer FC, Hofstetter SR, Liang HG, Coppa GF. Significant trends in the treatment of hepatic trauma: experience with 411 injuries. Ann Surg. 1992; 215:492–500.

[16] Shanmugana K, Mirvis SE. CT evaluation of the liver with acute blunt trauma. Crit Rev Diagn Imaging. 1995;36:73–113.

[17] Mirvis SE, Whitthey NO, Vainwright JR, Gens DR. Blunt hepatic trauma in adults: CT base classification and correlation with prognosis and treatment. Radiology 1989;171:27–32.

[18] Croce MA, Fabian TC, Kudsk KA, Baum SL, Payne LW, Mangiante LC, et al. AAST organ injury scale: correlation of CT graded liver injuries and operative findings. J Trauma. 1991;31(6):806–12.

[19] Yoon W, Jeong YY, Kim JK, Seo JJ, Lim HS, Shin SS, Kim JC, Jeong SW, Park JG, Kang HK. CT in blunt liver trauma. Radiographics. 2005; 25(1):87-104.
[20] Miele V, Andreoli C, de Cicco ML, Adami L, David V. Hemoperitoneum associated with liver bare area injuries: CT evaluation. Eur Radiol 2002; 12:765–769.
[21] Poletti PA, Mirvis SE, Shanmuganathan K, Killeen KL, Coldwell D. CT criteria for management of blunt liver trauma: correlation with angiographic and surgical findings. Radiology. 2000; 216:418–427.
[22] Hagiwara A, Murata A, Matsuda T, Matsuda H, Shimazaki S. The efficacy and limitations of transcatheter embolization for severe hepatic injury. J Trauma. 2002; 52:1091–1096.
[23] Fang JF, Chen RJ, Wong YC, et al. Pooling of contrast material on computed tomography mandates aggressive management of blunt hepatic injury. Am J Surg. 1998; 176:315–319.
[24] Fang JF, Chen RJ, Wong YC, et al. Classification and treatment of pooling of contrast material on computed tomographic scan of blunt hepatic trauma. J Trauma. 2000; 49:1083–1088.
[25] Wong YC, Wang LJ, See LC, et al. Contrast material extravasation on contrast-enhanced helical computed tomographic scan of blunt abdominal trauma: its significance on the choice, time, and outcome of treatment. J Trauma. 2003; 54:164– 170.
[26] Shanmuganathan K, Mirvis SE. CT scan evaluation of blunt hepatic trauma. Radiol Clin North Am. 1998; 36:399–41.
[27] Sica G, Bocchini G, Guida F, Tanga M, Guaglione M, Scaglione M. Multidetector computed tomography in the diagnosis and management of renal trauma. Radiol med. 2010; 115:936–949.
[28] Razali MR, Azian AA, Amran AR, Azlin S. Computed tomography of blunt renal trauma. Singapore Med J. 2010; 51(6): 468
[29] Lee YJ, oh SN , Rha SE, Byun JY. Renal trauma. Radiol clin Nam. 2007; (45): 581-592.
[30] Alonso RC, Borruel Nacenta S, Diez Martinez P, Guerrero AS, Fuentes CG. Kidney in Danger:CT Findings of Blunt and Penetrating Renal Trauma. RadioGraphics. 2009; 29: 2033–2053.
[31] Gupta A, Stuhlfaut JW, Fleming KW, Lucey BC, Soto JA. Blunt trauma of the pancreas and biliary tract: a multimodality imaging approach to diagnosis. Radiographics 2004; 24(5):1381-95.
[32] Linsenmaier U, Wirth S, Reiser M, Körner M. Diagnosis and classification of pancreatic and duodenal injuries in emergency radiology. Radiographics 2008; 28(6):1591-602.
[33] Cirillo RL Jr, Koniaris LG. Detecting blunt pancreatic injuries. J Gastrointest Surg. 2002; 6(4):587-9.
[34] Patel SV, Spencer JA, El-Hasani S, Sheridan MB. Imaging of pancreatic trauma. Br J Radiol. 1998; 71:985–990.
[35] Venkatesh SK, Chin Wan JM. CT of blunt pancreatic trauma–a pictorial essay. Eur J Radiol. 2008; 67:311–320.
[36] Shanmuganathan K. Multi-detector row CT imaging of blunt abdominal trauma. Semin Ultrasound CT MR. 2004; 25:180–204.

[37] Rekhi S, Anderson SW, Rhea JT, Soto JA. Imaging of blunt pancreatic trauma. Emerg Radiol. 2010;17(1):13-9. Epub 2009 Apr 25.
[38] Wong YC, Wang LJ, Lin BC et al. CT grading of blunt pancreatic injuries: prediction of ductal disruption and surgical correlation. J Comput Assist Tomogr. 1997; 21:246–250.
[39] Phelan HA, Velmahos GC et al. An evaluation of multidetector computed tomography in detecting pancreatic injury: results of a multicenter AAST study. J Trauma. 2009; 66(3):641-6; discussion 646-7.
[40] Lane MJ, Mindelzun RE, Sandhu JS et al. CT diagnosis of blunt pancreatic trauma: importance of detecting fluid between the pancreas and the splenic vein. AJR Am J Roentgenol. 1994; 163:833–835.
[41] Bradley EL, Young PR, Chang MC et al. Diagnosis and initial management of blunt pancreatic trauma: guidelines from a multiinstitutional review. Ann Surg. 1998; 227:861–869.
[42] Duchesne JC, Schmeig R, Islam S et al. Selective nonoperative management of low grade blunt pancreatic injury: are we there yet? J Trauma. 2008; 65:49–53.
[43] Brestas PS, Karakyklas D, Gardelis J et al. Sequential CT evaluation of isolated non-penetrating pancreatic trauma. JOP. 2006; 7:51–55.
[44] Anderson SW, Soto JA. Pancreatic duct evaluation: accuracy of portal venous phase 64 MDCT Abdom Imaging. 2009; 34:55–63.
[45] Wong YC, Wang LJ, Fang JF et al. Multidetector-row computed tomography (CT) of blunt pancreatic injuries: can contrast-enhanced multiphasic CT detect pancreatic duct injuries? J Trauma. 2008; 64:666–672.
[46] Kim HS, Lee DK, Kim IW, et al. The role of endoscopic retrograde pancreatography in the treatment of traumatic pancreatic duct injury. Gastrointest Endosc. 2001; 54:49–55.
[47] Ragozzino A, Manfredi R, Scaglione M et al. The use of MRCP in detection of pancreatic injuries after blunt trauma. Emerg Radiol. 2003; 10:14–18.
[48] Matos C, Winant C, Deviere J. Magnetic resonance pancreatography. Abdom Imaging. 2001; 26:243–253.
[49] Gillams AR, Kurzawinski T, Lees WR. Diagnosis of duct disruption and assessment of pancreatic leak with dynamic secretin-stimulated MR cholangiopancreatography. AJR Am J Roentgenol. 2006; 186:499–506.
[50] Broder J. Diagnostic Imaging for the Emergency Physician, 2011, p 578-611.
[51] McCullough CJ. Isolated mesenteric injury due to blunt abdominal trauma. Injury. 7, 295-298[5].
[52] Lassandro F, Romano S, Rossi G, Muto R, Cappabianca S, Grassi R. Gastric traumatic injuries: CT findings. Eur J Radiol. 2006; 59:349-54.
[53] Furuya Y, Yasuhara H, Ariki K, Yanagie H, Naka S, Nojiri T et al. Hepatic portal venous gas caused by blunt abdominal trauma: is it a true ominous sign of bowel necrosis? Report of a case. Surg Today. 2002; 32:655–8.
[54] Brody JM, Leighton DM, Murphy BL, Abbott GF, Vaccaro JP, Jagminas L, Cioffi WG. CT of blunt trauma bowel and mesenteric injury: typical findings and pitfalls in diagnosis. Radiographics. 2000; 20: 1525-36.

[55] Vu Nghiem H, Brooke Jeffrey R. Jr. and Mindelzun RE. CT of blunt trauma to the bowel and mesentery. AJR 1993; 160: 53 – 58.

[56] Brofman N, Atri M, Epid D, Hanson JM, Grinblat L, Chughtai T, Renneman F. Evaluation of Bowel and Mesenteric Blunt Trauma with Multidetector CT. RadioGraphics 2006; 26:1119–1131. .

[57] Nursal TZ, Ugurlu M, Kologlu M, Hamaloglu E. Traumatic diaphragmatic hernias: a report of 26 cases. Hernia 2001; 5: 25-91.

[58] Ramos CT, Koplewitz BZ, Babyn PS, Manson PS, Ein SH. What have we learned about traumatic diaphragmatic hernias in children? J Pediatr Surg 2000; 35:601-4.

[59] Sadeghi N, Nicaise N, DeBacker D, Struyven J, Van Gansbeke D. Right diaphragmatic rupture and hepatic hernia: an indirect sign on computed tomography. Eur Radiol 1999; 9:972-4.

[60] Eren S, Kantarci M, Okur A. Imaging of diaphragmatic rupture after trauma. Clin Radiol. 2006; 61(6):467-77.

[61] Nchimi A, Szapiro D, Ghaye B, Willems V, Khamis J, Haquet L, Noukoua C, Dondelinger RF. Helical CT of blunt diaphragmatic rupture. AJR Am J Roentgenol. 2005; 184(1):24-30.

[62] Chen HW, Wong YC, Wang LJ, Fu CJ, Fang JF, Lin BC. Computed tomography in left-sided and right-sided blunt diaphragmatic rupture: experience with 43 patients. Clin Radiol. 2010; 65(3):206-12. Epub 2010 Jan 4.

[63] Bergin D, Ennis R, Keogh C, Fenlon HM, Murray JG. The "dependent viscera" sign in CT diagnosis of blunt traumatic diaphragmatic. AJR Am J Roentgenol. 2001; 177(5):1137-40.

[64] Yoon W, Kim JK, Jeong YY, Seo JJ, Park JG, Kang HK. Pelvic arterial hemorrhage in patients with pelvic fractures: detection with contrast-enhanced CT. Radiographics. 2004; 24(6):1591-605.

[65] Shanmuganathan K, Mirvis SE, Sover ER. Value of contrast-enhanced CT in detecting active hemorrhage in patients with blunt abdominal or pelvic trauma. AJR Am J Roentgenol. 1993; 161:65-69.

[66] Cerva DS, Mirvis SE, Shanmuganathan K, Kelly IM, Pais SO. Detection of bleeding in patients with major pelvic fracture: value of contrast-enhanced CT. AJR Am J Roentgenol. 1996; 166:131–135.

[67] Stephen DJ, Kreder HJ, Day AC, et al. Early detection of arterial bleeding in acute pelvic trauma. J Trauma. 1999; 47:638–642.

[68] Pereira SJ, O'Brien DP, Luchette FA, et al. Dynamic helical computed tomography scan accurately detects hemorrhage in patients with pelvic fracture. Surgery. 2000; 128:678-685.

[69] Hagiwara A, Minakawa K, Fukushima H, Murata A, Masudo H, Shimazaki S. Predictors of death in patients with life-threatening pelvic hemorrhage after successful transcatheter arterial embolization. J Trauma. 2003; 55:696-703.

[70] Pereira SJ, O'Brien DP, Luchette FA, et al. Dynamic helical computed tomography scan accurately detects hemorrhage in patients with pelvic fracture. Surgery. 2000; 128:678–685.

[71] Pinto A, Niola R, Tortora G, Ponticiello G, Russo G, Di Nuzzo L, Gagliardi N, Scaglione M, Merola S, Stavolo C, Maglione F, Romano L. Role of multidetector-row CT in

assessing the source of arterial haemorrhage in patients with pelvic vascular trauma. Comparison with angiography. Radiol Med. 2010;115(4):648-67.
[72] Velmahos G, Toutouzas K, Vassiliu P, et al. A prospective study on the safety and efficacy of angiographic embolization for pelvic and visceral injuries. J Trauma 2002; 53:303-8.
[73] Kish J, Katz M, Marx M, Harrell D, Hanks S. N-butyl cyanoacrylate embolization for control of acute arterial hemorrhage. J Vasc Interv Radiol. 2004;15:689-95.
[74] Alonso M, Brathwaite C, Garcia V, et al. Practice management guidelines for the nonoperative management of blunt injury to the liver and spleen. In: www.east.org 2003.
[75] Haan J, Scott J, Boyd-Kranis R, Ho S, Kramer M, Scalea T. Admission angiography for blunt splenic injury: advantages and pitfalls. J Trauma. 2001; 51:1161-5.
[76] Bessoud B, Denys A. Main splenic artery embolization using coils in blunt splenic injuries: Effects on the intrasplenic blood pressure. Eur Radiol. 2004; 14:1718-9.
[77] Velmahos G, Toutouzas K, Radin R, Cjan L, Demetriades D. Nonoperative treatment of blunt injury to solid abdominal organs. J Trauma 2003;138:844-51.
[78] Hagiwara A, Yukioka T, Ohta S, et al. Nonsurgical management of patients with blunt hepatic injury: efficacy of transcatheter arterial embolization. AJR 1997;169:1151-6.
[79] Velmahos G, Toutouzas K, Radin R, Cjan L, Demetriades D. Nonoperative treatment of blunt injury to solid abdominal organs. J Trauma. 2003; 138:844-5.
[80] Dinkel H, Danuse RH, Triller J. Blunt renal trauma: minimally invasive management with microcatheter embolization experience in nine patients. Radiology 2002; 223:723-30.
[81] Cook R, Keating J, Gillespie I. The role of angiography in the management of haemorrhage from major fractures of the pelvis. J Bone Joint Surg Br. 2002; 84:178-82.
[82] Nance FC, Wennar MH, Johnson LW, Ingram JC Jr, Cohn I Jr. Surgical judgment in the management of penetrating wounds of the abdomen: experience with 2212 patients. Ann Surg. 1974; 179(5): 639–646.
[83] Lowe RJ, Saletta JD, Read DR, Radhakrishnan J, Moss GS. Should laparotomy be mandatory or selective in gunshot wounds of the abdomen? J Trauma. 1977; 17(12): 903–907.
[84] Renz BM, Feliciano DV. Unnecessary laparotomies for trauma: a prospective study of morbidity. J Trauma. 1995; 38 (3):350–356.
[85] Henderson VJ, Organ CH Jr, Smith RS. Negative trauma celiotomy. Am Surg. 1993; 59(6):365–370.

Section 2

Techniques of Anesthesia in Abdominal Surgery

Chapter 2

Anesthetic Management of Abdominal Surgery

Aysin Alagol

Additional information is available at the end of the chapter

http://dx.doi.org/10.5772/49940

1. Introduction

General or regional anesthesia can be appropriate for patients undergoing abdominal surgery. In common practice, balanced anesthesia with inhalational anesthetics, opioids and neuromuscular blockers are used in general anesthesia for abdominal surgical procedures. Endotracheal intubation as well as Laryngeal Mask Airway can be used for airway control. Regional anesthesia, mainly central blocks, can be used either as a sole anesthetic technique or combined with general anesthesia. Effective sedation is indicated when regional techniques were used alone. There are few absolute contraindications of spinal and epidural anesthesia including patient refusal and raised intracranial pressure. Relative contraindications are administration of anticoagulants, skin or tissue infections at the proposed site of needle insertion, severe hypovolemia and lack of anesthesiologist's experience. Postoperative headache after spinal may make epidural technique preferred, or, duration of the surgical procedure may be so short that spinal anesthesia may be more practical than epidural, need for prolonged postoperative analgesia makes catheter technique preferred than single-shot technique, etc. (1).

2. Problems associated with abdominal surgery

Pulmonary function is impaired after abdominal surgery more severely than after non-thoracic, non-abdominal surgery. Upper abdominal procedures result in a higher incidence of pulmonary complications. Postoperative pain control improves the pattern and effectiveness of ventilation provided that excessive sedation and depression of ventilation should be avoided. Epidural-subarachnoid administration of opioids or patient-controlled analgesia is recommended for postoperative pain management.

Heat loss via radiation, conduction and evaporation is a particular problem during abdominal surgery. As heat loss causes decreased organ perfusion and metabolic acidosis, and can not be avoided, all fluids including skin preparation, irrigation and intravenous fluids should be warmed. Heated mattress should be used. Anesthesia circuits should be humidified. Low-flow or closed circuit technique is recommended.

Mechanical bowel preparation, laxatives, ileostomies, preoperative vomiting and/or diarrhoea, when present, cause large fluid loses in patients undergoing abdominal surgery. Intraoperative ascites removal is not associated with hypotension untill translocation of fluids continues or intravascular volume is not maintained (2).

Patients with cancer may have perioperative complications related to the disease or therapy. In patients with colon, pancreas and stomach cancer, hypercoagulability is common. Previous chemotherapy can cause anemia, renal, hepatic and pulmonary toxicity and, cardiomyopaty. Chronic opioid therapy for cancer pain requires greater doses of opioids for postoperative pain management (2).

3. Preoperative evaluation

The purpose of preoperative evaluation is to obtain current and previous medical status. It will give us ability of perioperative patient management. As medical problems can affect anesthesia, anesthesiologist should have knowledge about and manage them perioperatively. Then perioperative comfort can be reached: reduced patient anxiety, decrease of delays of surgery, less postoperative morbidity etc..

Preoperative risk assessment is performed by using ASA risk classification system which was developed in 1941 (Table 1). The system was based on the patients preoperative medical conditions and neither the type of anesthesia nor the type of surgery was considered in this classification. Preoperative physical examination should include, at least, blood pressure, heart rate, respiratory rate, height and weight. BMI can be calculated. The evaluation of the airway includes inspecting the teeth and measuring length and range of motion of the neck, thyromental distance and Mallampati classification which is performed by asking patients open the mouth widely (Table 2). Auscultation of the heart and lungs; observing the patient's effort for walking, can predict the need for further testing. For patients with risk factors for coronary artery disease, or who have symptoms of ischemia, an ECG is indicated.

Morbidly obese patients have higher incidence of difficult tracheal intubation, decreased oxgnenation, increased gastric volume, pulmonary embolism and sudden death. Heart disease, hypertension and Obstructive Sleep Apnea (OSA) are more common in obese patients. Obesity, hypertension and large neck circumference (>60cm) predict OSA. This neck measurement also predicts difficult ventilation and intubation.

Preoperative diagnostic and laboratory evaluation depends on the patient's medical status and history and the surgical procedures. The requirement of complete blood count, liver function, renal function and coagulation testings, urinanalysis, chest radiography in patients undergoing abdominal surgery is similar with other surgical procedures (3).

ASA 1	Healthy patient without organic, biochemical, or psychiatric disease.
ASA 2	A patient with mild systemic disease e.g., mild asthma or well controlled hypertension. No significant impact on daily activity. Unlikely to have an impact on anesthesia and surgery.
ASA 3	Significant or severe systemic disease that limits normal activity, e.g., renal failure on dialysis or class II congestive heart failure. Significant impact on daily activity. Probable impact on anesthesia and surgery.
ASA 4	Severe disease that is a constant threat to life or requires intensive therapy, e.g., acute myocardial infarction, respiratory failure requiring mechanical ventilation. Major impact on anesthesia and surgery.
ASA 5	Moribund patient who is equally likely to die in the next 24 hours with or without surgery.
ASA 6	Brain-dead organ donor

'E' added indicates emergency surgery

Table 1. American Society of Anesthesiologists Physical Status Classification

Class I	The soft palate, fauces, entire uvula, and pillars are visualized
Class II	The soft palate, fauces, and a portion of the uvula are visualized
Class III	The soft palate and base of the uvula are visualized
Class IV	The hard palate only is visualized

Table 2. Mallampati Classification

3.1. Preoperative evaluation of patients with cardiovascular disorders

The most common perioperative cardiovascular problem is hypertension which can be defined as blood pressure (BP) greater than 140/90 mmHg. It is recommended to delay elective surgery for Systolic BP>200 mmHg and Diastolic BP>115 mmHg. In the presence of ischemic heart disease, Revised Cardiac Risk Index has been validated as the best to predict perioperative cardiac risk (Table 3). In patients with heart failure, anesthesiologist should focus on minimizing the effects of the disease preoperatively. Decompensated heart failure is a high risk condition and is an indication for delaying elective surgery. Medical therapy of hypertension and other cardiac diseases should be continued preoperatively, and should be administered on the day of surgery. In patients with mitral stenosis, heart rate should be controlled prior to surgery. Beta-blockers are used and continued until the day of surgery to control atrial fibrillation. On the other hand, chronic mitral regurgitation is usually well tolerated perioperatively. In the presence of mitral valve prolapse, it is necessary to diagnose if there is significant valve degeneration. Aortic stenosis increases risk of bleeding and, patients with severe stenosis should be evaluated by cardiologist preoperatively. Aortic insufficiency is generally well tolerated and has low risks of anesthesia. Prophylaxis for infective endocarditis is no longer recommended in valvular diseases. Some rhythm abnormalities such as isolated right bundle branch block is not a risk factor for anesthesia, but as left bundle branch block is associated with coronary artery disease, it is more important for anesthesiologist. For patients with rapid ventricular rated atrial fibrillation, preoperative rate control-with β-blockers is recommended. If ventricular arrhytmias are benign (isolated ventricular premature beats, VPB) there is no risk perioperatively, but, if VPBs >30/hour, it is potencially lethal.

1. Criteria
1. High Risk Surgery: 1 Point
2. Coronary Artery Disease: 1 Point
3. Congestive Heart Failure: 1 Point
4. Cerebrovascular Disease: 1 Point
5. Diabetes Mellitus on Insulin: 1 Point
6. Serum Creatinine >2 mg/dl: 1 Point
2. Interpretation
1. Scoring
1. Points 0: Class I Very Low (0.4% complications)
2. Points 1: Class II Low (0.9% complications)
3. Points 2: Class III Moderate (6.6% complications)
4. Points 3: Class IV High (>11% complications)
2. Complications predicted by above scoring
1. Myocardial Infarction
2. Pulmonary Embolism
3. Ventricular Fibrillation
4. Cardiac Arrest
5. Complete Heart Block

Table 3. Revised Cardiac Risk Index

3.2. Preoperative evaluation of patients with pulmonary risks

Asthma, if well-controlled, provides less risk for complications. Pulmonary function tests are indicated only in diagnosis or assessment of therapy, and not for risk assessment. Risks for pulmonary complications include smoking, age>70 years, ASA score>2, prolonged surgery (>2 hours), chronic obstructive pulmonary disease (COPD), BMI>30, hypoalbuminemia (<3 g/dL). Alternatives to general anesthesia such as epidural anesthesia may provide less postoperative pulmonary complications.

3.3. Preoperative evaluation of patients with hepatic disorders

In case of history of hepatitis, it is important whether acute episode occured soon after surgery. Elective surgery is contraindicated in patients with acute disease. Severe liver disease cause high perioperative morbidity and mortality. This can be predicted by using the Child-Turcotte-Pugh classification (Table 4). The cause and the degree of hepatic dysfunction are important (3).

Parameter	1	2	3
Ascites	Absent	Slight	Moderate
Bilirubin (mg/dL)	<2	2-3	>3
Albumin (g/dL)	<3.5	2.8-3.5	<2.8
Prothrombin Time (sec)	<4	4-6	>6
Encephalopathy	none	Grade 1-2	Grade 3-4

Table 4. Child-Turcotte-Pugh Classification

3.4. Drugs and alternative therapies

Although there are no official standards or guidelines on the preoperative use of herbal medications, it is suggested that herbals be discontinued at lest 2-3 weeks before surgery. On the other hand, in practice, anesthesiologists cannot evaluate patients 2-3 weeks before surgery. Therefore, anesthesiologists should be familiar with herbals, their complications and treatments (4).

3.5. Preoperative evaluation of morbidly obese patients

Obesity is associated with increased risk of cardiovascular diseases and diabetes mellitus. Obstructive sleep apnea (OSA) and cancer are more common in obese patients. Then, preoperative evaluation should be focused on coexisting diseases as well as on airway, history of snoring, and vital signs. Neck circumference should be measured. Patients with OSA should bring their continuous positive airway pressure devices to the hospital to use postoperatively.

3.6. Preoperative fasting

The main indication of preoperative fasting recommendation is to reduce risk of pulmonary aspiration. The ASA guideline supports a fasting period of 2 hours for clear liquids. A fasting period of 6 hours after a light meal and 8 hours after a meal that includes fried or fatty foods is recommended (5). Solid food should be prohibited for 6 h before elective surgery in adults and children, although patients should not have their operation cancelled or delayed just because they are chewing gum, sucking a boiled sweet or smoking immediately prior to induction of anaesthesia. These recommendations also apply to patients with obesity and gastro-oesophageal reflux (6). Preoperatively administered carbohydrate-rich drink can reduce discomfort during the period of waiting before elective surgery compared with preoperative oral intake of water or overnight fasting (7).

4. Hepatic function and anesthesia

Anesthetics and surgical procedure can induce hepatic function; on the other hand, hepatic dysfunction can impair the response to anesthesia and surgery. Influence of volatile anesthetics on hepatic blood flow and function is related not only tothe anesthetic itself but also to the severity of hepatic dysfunction and abdominal surgical maniplation. Volatile anesthetics affect hepatic blood flow. Some other conditions may influence hepatic blood flow including age, volemia, intraoperative position, surgical procedure, blood pressure changes, local anesthetics, vasopressors, hemoglobin level and arterial oxygen concentrations. Anesthetics decrease cardiac output and then decrease portal blood flow; but they may increase hepatic arterial blood flow. Total hepatic flow can be restored, but often normal values can not be reached. Volatile anesthetics alter portal venous and hepatic arterial vascular resistance. Sevoflurane maintains hepatic arterial blood flow and hepatic O_2 delivery. Compound A does not alter hepatic function. No clinical hepatotoxicity has been found by using low and high flow sevoflurane and isoflurane anesthesia. In patients with chronic liver disease, isoflurane and desflurane have not changed liver function tests. Indeed, xenon seems to be the ideal anesthetic gas as it appears to be having no effect on organ perfusion; no changes on hepatic arterial blood flow. Intravenous anesthetics can affect hepatic function; thiopental and etomidate decrease hepatic blood flow, propofol increases portal and hepatic arterial blood flow. But intravenous anesthetics have not demonstrated significant effect on postoperative liver function. The effect of central neuroaxial blocks on liver function is still unclear.

Abdominal surgery reduces total hepatic blood flow. Pneumoperitoneum can increase hepatic perfusion during CO_2 insuflation. Surgical operations of biliary tract, colon, stomach and, hepatic resection for HCC are risk factors for perioperative hepatic failure. Perioperative hemorrhage is common in patients with preoperative hepatic dysfunction.

5. Anesthetic management of hepatic resection

It is important to diagnose the presence of esophageal varices. In case of thrombocytopenia, those large esophageal varices are major perioperative risk factors. Coagulopathy and anemia should be corrected prior to surgery. There is a significant risk of bleeding intraoperatively. Invasive monitoring and ability of rapid transfusion i.e. venous access- is essential. Intravenous fluids should be supplemented with sodium and potassium. The severity of liver failure and majority of hepatic resection affect the choice and dosing of anesthetic drugs as well as postoperative pain treatment (8).

6. Anesthetic management of abdominal organ transplantation

Except living donor recipients, these cases are accepted as emergency cases. Patients undergoing liver transplantation should be evaluated by multiple medical specialists. Medical and physical examinations should be done carefully. But, as the patients wait long time for transplantation, changes could have occurred since the last evaluation. The patient may have pulmonary hypertension, then pulmonary artery catheterisation is needed and can be performed preoperatively, i.e, in the ICU. The prevalence of cardiac disease is greater in liver transplant patients than in the general public. Complications of cardiac disease play a large role in early mortality and graft loss in the postoperative period. While the presence of risk factors seems to predict coronary disease in renal disease, these factors do not perform as well in liver disease. Intraoperative monitoring may include transesophageal echocardiography also. In the preoperative period, red blood cells, fresh frozen plasma (10 U each) must be ready and 4 Units of platelets available (9,10).

General anesthesia induction and maintenance is nearly similar with any other surgery. Atracurium or cisatracurium is preferred to vecuronium, because atracurium is independent of liver for clerance. If neuromuscular monitoring is performed, any muscle relaxant can be used. An arterial line and central venous line are necessary and, ultrasound can be used to facilitate the access. As these patients are hypovolemic and have low peripheral resistance, induction of anesthesia can cause severe hypotension. After induction, an orogastric or nasogastric tube should be placed for gastric decompression. As patients have coagulopathy, placement of nasogastric tube can cause severe bleeding. Optimal anesthetic technique has not been defined for maintenance of anesthesia. Volatile anesthetics are suitable for liver transplantation, except halothane. Balanced technique using volatile agent and opioids, or total intravenous anesthesia using benzodiazepines and opioids can be used, with oxgen in air and without Nitrous oxyde for liver transplantation.

Peroperative hypothermia should be treated by blankets and warm intravenous fluids. Some tests are necessary during intraoperative period; arterial blood gase analysis, hematocrit, blood glucose and electrolytes.

There are three phases of liver transplantation; dissection, anhepatic and neo-hepatic phases. During dissection, hypotension frequently develops and adequate fluid replacement and management of diuresis are crucial.

Acidosis and hypocalemia frequently occur during the anhepatic stage. During early reperfusion phase, severe hemodynamic changes and cardiac arrest can ocur when the vascular clamps are removed. Coagulopathy or bleeding can develop in the reperfusion phase. Hypertension may occur during abdominal closure.

After liver transplantation, patients can be extubated in the operating room (11-14). On the other hand, close monitoring and laboratory tests have to be continued in the ICU. Patients undergoing liver transplantation have decreased analgesic requirements when compared with other major abdominal surgery; it was concluded that orthotopic liver transplant patients experienced less pain and used less morphine postoperatively than did liver resection patients (15).

7. Anesthetic management of laparoscopic surgery

Laparoscopy was used for gynecologic diagnostic procedures in 1970s. Then, in 1980s, laparoscopic cholecystectomies were started (16). Although physiologic changes during this procedure can complicate anesthetic management, absolute contraindications are rare.

The routine pneumoperitoneum technique for laparoscopy is insufflation of CO_2. CO_2 is more soluble in blood than air, O_2 and N_2O. Pneumoperitoneum results in ventilatory and respiratory changes. First, pneumoperitoneum decreases thoracopulmonary compliance and, elevation of diaphragm can cause atelectasis, ventilation-perfusion changes can occur. $PaCO_2$ increases from the beginning of insufflation and, reaches maximum at 15-30th minute in patients undergoing laparoscopic cholecystectomy under head up position. After this period, increase in $PaCO_2$ requires a search for another cause. $PaCO_2$ increases more in ASA class II and III patients than in ASA I patients. The main cause of increased $PaCO_2$ is absorption of CO_2 from peritoneum, and the second, hypoventilation caused by abdominal distension, position, or volume-controlled mechanical ventilation. Increased $PaCO_2$ can be corrected by a %10-25 increase in alveolar ventilation. During pneumoperitoneum, endotracheal tube can move into bronchi because of cephalad displacement of diaphragm. Anesthesiologist should be aware of increased plateau airway pressure to notice endobronchial intubation (17).

Intraoperative standard monitoring should include arterial blood pressure, heart rate, electrocardiograpy, pulse oximetry, capnometry, and, in case of severe heart disease, transeosephageal echocardiography in laparoscopic procedures. Endotracheal intubation and controlled ventilation is the safest anesthetic technique. The laryngeal mask airway (LMA) has been used as an alternative to tracheal intubation but, aspiration of gastric contens may occur. The Proseal LMA is a more effective ventilatory device for laparoscopic cholecystectomy than LMA and the use of LMA for laparoscopic cholecystectomy is not recommended (18). Use of NO_2 is not contrindicated for laparoscopic cholecystectomy, but would be better to use air instead of NO_2 during intestinal or colonic procedures (19,20). Deep muscle relaxation is desirable, but is not clear that it is obliged. The choice of anesthetic drug does not play a direct role in patient outcome. As mask ventilation inflates the stomach during induction, an orogastric /nasogastric tube placement and aspiration before trochar placement is necessary. During pneumoperitoneum, $PETCO_2$ must be maintained between 35-40 mmHg. Intraoperative patient tilt should not exceed 15-20 degrees and positioning must be slow to avoid hemodynamic changes. Inflation and deflation should be done slowly. Peritoneal insufflation induces hemodynamic changes such as decreases in cardiac output independent of head-down or head-tilt position of patient, elevated arterial and systemic/pulmonary vascular resistances. Heart rate may increase slightly but, reflex increases of vagal tone can cause bradycardia or, even asystole. Then, atropine should be available. Intracranial pressure rises during pneumoperitoneum. These hemodynamic changes seem to be similar in high-risk cardiac patients and healthy patients qualitatively, but not quantitatively. Severe heart failure and terminal valvular insufficiency are more important than ischemic heart disease in being prone to cardiac complications during laparoscopic procedures. Vasodilators, α-2 agonists and remifentanil infusions are preferred to reduce the hemodynamic changes, especially in cardiac patients. In patients with chronic obstructive pulmonary disease (COPD), increased respiratory rate is a beter choice than increased tidal volume (17).

Postoperatively, O_2 should be administered after laparoscopic surgery. Nausea and vomiting is one of important postoperative morbidity after laparoscopic surgery and should be prevented and/or treated by using antiemetics (21,22).

Although general anesthesia with endotracheal intubation and controlled ventilation is the most frequently used anesthetic technique, regional anesthesia can be used safely for laparoscopic procedures. Epidural technique reduces opioid use, provides better muscular relaxation, shorter duration in recovery room, but, on the other hand, discomfort or shoulder pain caused by abdominal distention cannot be completely alleviated with epidural anesthesia and/or analgesia (23-25). Spinal anesthesia has been used only contemplated in patients where general anesthesia is contraindicated for laparoscopic cholecystectomy, however, a study in 3492 patients has found a number of advantages of spinal anesthesia, and it was concluded that spinal anesthesia should be the anesthesia of choice (26). This result was supported by recent studies, moreover the cost of spinal anesthesia has been found lower than that of general anesthesia (27). Regional anesthesia provides decreased PONV and hemodynamic changes and quicker recovery, it also requires gentle surgical manipulation, otherwise may cause anxiety and discomfort.

The most dangerous complication of laparoscopic procedures is gas embolism. It occurs mainly during the induction of insufflation. Intravascular injection of gas or, insufflation into an abdominal organ cause gas embolism. In addition to gas in vena cava and right atrium which causes a sudden fall in cardiac output, foramen ovale can open and a paradoxal embolism may ocur. Clinical findings depend on the volume of the embolus. If the volume is less than 0.5 ml/kg of air, embolism can be detected by invasive monitors without clinical signs; pulmonary artery pressure increases and doppler sounds changes. If the volume is 2 mL/kg of air, typical clinical symptom and signs appear; hypotension, tachycardia, cyanosis, arrhythmias, increased central venous pressure, and auscultation of millwheel murmur, decreased $PETCO_2$ and increased gradient between $PaCO_2$ and $PETCO_2$ (Δa-$PETCO_2$). When diagnosed, first insufflation should be stopped and pneumoperitoneum should be released for treatment of gas embolism. Patient should immediately be placed into head-down + left lateral decubitus position and hyperventilation with %100 O_2 should be reached. Aspiration of gas from central venous catheter is both diagnostic and therapeutic. In prevention of gas embolism, volume preload can be effective.

7.1. Postoperative pain management

Laparoscopy provides reduction in postoperative pain and analgesic consumption when compared with laparotomy. The nature of pain is also different; pain after laparotomy is parietal, mainly in the abdominal wall, on the other hand, pain after laparoscopic cholecystectomy is multifactorial. Visceral pain is common, but, port site local anesthetic infiltration provides analgesia. Non-steroidal antiinflammatory drugs (NSAID) are effective for pain relief after laparoscopic procedures (17).

In a recent study, bilateral ultrasound-guided TAP block has been found equivalent to local anesthetic infiltration of trocar insertion sites for overall postoperative pain in 80 patients undergoing laparoscopic cholecystectomy (28).

8. Anesthetic management of bariatric surgery

Obese patients have co-morbidities as hypertension, obstructive sleep apnoea, obesity-hypoventilation syndrome, non-alcoholic fatty liver disease and diabetes mellitus. Thus, these patients frequently need ICU after surgery. Airway management can be difficult in obese patients caused by short neck, pharyngeal soft tissue, large tongue; although BMI was not found to be associated with intubation difficulties in a study (29). Obese patients can have decreased lung capacities and are prone to undergo rapid oxygen desaturation. Morbid obesity is associated with a reduction in time to desaturate during apnoea following standard pre-oxygenation and induction of anaesthesia (30). During induction of general anesthesia, CPAP can be added to preoxygenation to prevent atelectasis. The volume of distribution of lipophilic drugs is changed in obese patients, except remifentanil. Induction dose of propofol, and, rocuronium, vecuronium and remifentanil should be dosed by using ideal body weight (IBW); thiopental, benzodiazepines, maintenance dose of propofol, atracurium, succinylcholine, fentanyl and sufentanyl can be dosed by using total body weight (TBW) (31,32). Reverse Trendelenburg position is an appropriate intraoperative position for obese patients because it causes minimal arterial blood pressure changes and improves oxygenation (33). As obese patients seem to be having more frequent complications caused by intraoperative positions, further care is needed during positioning. During pneumoperitoneum pulmonary resistance increases. Alveolar recruitment by repeated lung inflation to 50 mmHg or with vital capacity maneuver followed mechanical ventilation with PEEP 10-12 cmH_2O, and beach chair position has been effective at preventing lung atelectasis and is associated with better oxygenation in obese patients undergoing laparoscopic bariatric surgery (34-37). In addition to pneumoperitoneum, body mass is an important determinant of respiratory function during anaesthesia in obese patients. The recruitment maneuver should always be performed when a volemic and hemodynamic stabilisation is reached after induction of anaesthesia.

In the postoperative period, beach chair position, aggressive physiotherapy, noninvasive respiratory support and short-term recovery in critical care units with care of fluid management and pain may reduce pulmonary complications. Postoperative analgesia can be provided by intravenous or thoracic epidural Patient Controlled Analgesia. Non-opioids reduce opioid consumption and side effects (29).

9. Enhanced recovery after surgery

Enhanced Recovery After Surgery (ERAS) is a multimodal perioperative care pathway designed to achieve early recovery for patients undergoing major surgery. Initiated by Professor Henrik Kehlet in the 1990s, ERAS or "fast-track" programs have become an important focus of perioperative management after colorectal surgery (38,39).

The factors which delay going home after major GI surgery are; pain, lack of gastrointestinal function and immobility. Therefore postoperative management should include pain control, to promote gastrointestinal function and mobility as soon as possible (40,41).

ERAS is associated with more rapid recovery and shortened length of stay more than 30% and appears to be associated with reduced post-operative complications up to 50% (40).

Anesthesiologist has a role in ERAS as well as surgeon. Patients should not receive sedative premedication, long-acting opioids should be avoided, mid-thoracic epidural anaesthesia can be preferred. Avoidance of fluid overload and the use of body warmers for maintenance of normothermia intraoperatively are recommended. Prevention of postoperative nausea and vomiting should be induced (42).

Postoperative care should include continuous epidural mid-thoracic low-dose local anaesthetic and opioid combinations for approximately 48 hours following elective colonic surgery and approximately 96 hours following pelvic surgery. Acetaminophen (paracetamol) should be used as a baseline analgesic (4 g/day) throughout the post-operative course. For breakthrough pain, epidural boluses should be given while the epidural is running. Nonsteroidal anti-inflammatory drugs should be started at removal of the epidural catheter. Nasogastric tubes should not be used routinely in the postoperative period, and, oral nutritional supplements should be prescribed from the day of surgery until normal food intake is achieved.

A care plan that facilitates patients being out of bed for 2 hours on the day of surgery - followed by 6 hours - is recommended as early mobilisation. Stimulation of gut motility is also recommended.

In summary, the core principles of ERAS are to minimise invasive surgery and optimise pain control, and gastrointestinal function; less intravenous fluids, taking solid foods and fluids, and early mobilisation. And the goal of ERAS is not to decrease hospital stay but to enhance recovery, perioperative organ dysfunction and morbidity (43).

Author details

Aysin Alagol
Anesthesiology and Reanimation Clinic, Bagcilar Educational Hospital, Istanbul, Turkey

10. References

[1] D.L. Brown. Spinal, Epidural, and Caudal Anesthesia . In:Miller's Anesthesia. 7th ed. Ed.:R. D. Miller, L. I. Eriksson, L. A. Fleisher, J.P. Wiener-Kronish, W. Young. Churchill Livingstone, Philadelphia.Vol 2.pp:1611-1638.

[2] Bjoraker D.G. Abdominal and Major vascular Surgery.In:Anaesthesia.Editors: W.S. Nimmo, G. Smith, Blackwell Scientific Publications, Oxford. Vol 1, pp: 726-744.

[3] S.P.Fischer, A.M.Bader, B.J.Sweizer. Preoperative Evaluation. In:Miller's Anesthesia. 7th ed. Ed.:R. D. Miller, L. I. Eriksson, L. A. Fleisher, J.P. Wiener-Kronish, W. Young. Churchill Livingstone, Philadelphia.Vol 1.pp:1001-1066.

[4] M.A.Lee, C.S. Yuan, J. Moss. Complementary and Alternative Therapies. In:Miller's Anesthesia. 7th ed. Ed.:R. D. Miller, L. I. Eriksson, L. A. Fleisher, J.P. Wiener-Kronish, W. Young. Churchill Livingstone, Philadelphia.Vol 1.pp: 957-966.

[5] ASA Practice Guidelines for Preoperative Fasting and the Use of Pharmacologic Agents to Reduce the Risk of Pulmonary Aspiration: Application to Healthy Patients Undergoing Elective Procedures: An Updated Report by the American Society of Anesthesiologists Committee on Standards and Practice Parameters. Anesthesiology: March 2011 - Volume 114 - Issue 3 - pp 495-511.

[6] Smith I, Kranke P, Murat I, Smith A, O'Sullivan G, Søreide E, Spies C, in't Veld B; European Society of Anaesthesiology. Perioperative fasting in adults and children: guidelines from the European Society of Anaesthesiology. Eur J Anaesthesiol. 2011 Aug;28(8):556-69.

[7] Hausel J, Nygren J, Lagerkranser M, Hellström PM, Hammarqvist F, Almström C, Lindh A, Thorell A, Ljungqvist O. A carbohydrate-rich drink reduces preoperative discomfort in elective surgery patients. Anesth Analg. 2001 Nov;93(5):1344-50.

[8] D.M.Rothenberg, C.J.O'Connor, K.J.Tuman. Anesthesia and the Hepatobiliary System. In:Miller's Anesthesia. 7th ed. Ed.:R. D. Miller, L. I. Eriksson, L. A. Fleisher, J.P. Wiener-Kronish, W. Young. Churchill Livingstone, Philadelphia.Vol 1.pp: 2135-53.

[9] C.S. Yost and C.U.Niemann. Anesthesia for Abdominal Organ Transplantation. In: Miller's Anesthesia. 7th ed. Ed.:R. D. Miller, L. I. Eriksson, L. A. Fleisher, J.P. Wiener-Kronish, W. Young. Churchill Livingstone, Philadelphia.Vol 1.pp: 2155-2184.

[10] Findlay JY, Wen D, Mandell MS. Cardiac risk evaluation for abdominal transplantation. Curr Opin Organ Transplant. 2010 Jun;15(3): 363-367.

[11] Glanemann M, Langrehr J, Kaisers U, Schenk R, Müller A, Stange B, Neumann U, Bechstein WO, Falke K, Neuhaus P. Postoperative tracheal extubation after orthotopic liver transplantation. Acta Anaesthesiol Scand. 2001 Mar;45(3): 333-339.

[12] Neelakanta G, Sopher M, Chan S, Pregler J, Steadman R, Braunfeld M, Csete M. Early tracheal extubation after liver transplantation. J Cardiothorac Vasc Anesth. 1997 Apr;11(2): 165-167.

[13] Mandell MS, Lezotte D, Kam I, Zamudio S. Reduced use of intensive care after liver transplantation: patient attributes that determine early transfer to surgical wards. Liver Transpl. 2002 Aug;8(8): 682-687.

[14] Mandell MS, Stoner TJ, Barnett R, Shaked A, Bellamy M, Biancofiore G, Niemann C, Walia A, Vater Y, Tran ZV, Kam I. A multicenter evaluation of safety of early extubation in liver transplant recipients. Liver Transpl. 2007 Nov;13(11): 1557-1563.

[15] Moretti EW, Robertson KM, Tuttle-Newhall JE, Clavien PA, Gan TJ. Orthotopic liver transplant patients require less postoperative morphine than do patients undergoing hepatic resection. J Clin Anesth. 2002 Sep;14(6): 416-412.

[16] Dubois F, Icard P, Berthelot G, Levard H. Coelioscopic cholecystectomy. Preliminary report of 36 cases. Ann Surg. 1990 Jan;211(1): 60-62.

[17] J.L.Joris. Anesthesia for Laparoscopic Surgery. In: Miller's Anesthesia. 7th ed. Ed.:R. D. Miller, L. I. Eriksson, L. A. Fleisher, J.P. Wiener-Kronish, W. Young. Churchill Livingstone, Philadelphia.Vol 1.pp: 2185-2202.

[18] Lu PP, Brimacombe J, Yang C, Shyr M. ProSeal versus the Classic laryngeal mask airway for positive pressure ventilation during laparoscopic cholecystectomy. Br J Anaesth. 2002 Jun;88(6): 824-827.

[19] Taylor E, Feinstein R, White PF, Soper N. Anesthesia for laparoscopic cholecystectomy. Is nitrous oxide contraindicated? Anesthesiology. 1992 Apr;76(4): 541-543.

[20] Akca O, Lenhardt R, Fleischmann E, Treschan T, Greif R, Fleischhackl R, Kimberger O, Kurz A, Sessler DI. Nitrous oxide increases the incidence of bowel distension in patients undergoing elective colon resection. Acta Anaesthesiol Scand. 2004 Aug;48(7): 894-898.

[21] Brindle GF, Soliman MG. Anaesthetic complications in surgical out-patients Can Anaesth Soc J. 1975 Sep;22(5): 613-619.

[22] Wu SJ, Xiong XZ, Cheng TY, Lin YX, Cheng NS.Efficacy of Ondansetron vs. Metoclopramide in Prophylaxis of Postoperative Nausea and Vomiting after Laparoscopic Cholecystectomy: A Systematic Review and Meta-Analysis. Hepatogastroenterology. 2012 Jan 20;59(119). doi: 10.5754/hge11811.

[23] Zhang HW, Chen YJ, Cao MH, Ji FT. Laparoscopic cholecystectomy under epidural anesthesia: a retrospective comparison of 100 patients. Am Surg. 2012 Jan;78(1): 107-110.

[24] Gramatica L Jr, Brasesco OE, Mercado Luna A, Martinessi V, Panebianco G, Labaque F, Rosin D, Rosenthal RJ, Gramatica L. Laparoscopic cholecystectomy performed under regional anesthesia in patients with chronic obstructive pulmonary disease. Surg Endosc. 2002 Mar;16(3): 472-475. Epub 2001 Nov 30.

[25] Chilvers CR, Vaghadia H, Mitchell GW, Merrick PM. Small-dose hypobaric lidocaine-fentanyl spinal anesthesia for short duration outpatient laparoscopy. II. Optimal fentanyl dose. Anesth Analg. 1997 Jan;84(1): 65-70.

[26] Sinha R, Gurwara AK, Gupta SC. Laparoscopic cholecystectomy under spinal anesthesia: a study of 3492 patients. J Laparoendosc Adv Surg Tech A. 2009 Jun;19(3):323-7. Laparoscopic cholecystectomy under spinal anesthesia: a study of 3492 patients.

[27] Liu X, Wei C, Wang Z, Wang H. Different anesthesia methods for laparoscopic cholecystectomy .Anaesthesist. 2011 Aug;60(8):723-8. Epub 2011 Feb 26.

[28] Ortiz J, Suliburk JW, Wu K, Bailard NS, Mason C, Minard CG, Palvadi RR. Bilateral transversus abdominis plane block does not decrease postoperative pain after laparoscopic cholecystectomy when compared with local anesthetic infiltration of trocar insertion sites. Reg Anesth Pain Med. 2012 Mar;37(2): 188-192.

[29] Brodsky JB, Lemmens HJ, Brock-Utne JG, Vierra M, Saidman LJ. Morbid obesity and tracheal intubation. Anesth Analg. 2002 Mar;94(3):732-6.

[30] A.C.Sinha and D.M.Eckman. Anesthesia for Bariatric Surgery. In: Miller's Anesthesia. 7th ed. Ed.:R. D. Miller, L. I. Eriksson, L. A. Fleisher, J.P. Wiener-Kronish, W. Young. Churchill Livingstone, Philadelphia.Vol 1.pp: 2089-2104.

[31] Egan TD, Huizinga B, Gupta SK, Jaarsma RL, Sperry RJ, Yee JB, Muir KT. Remifentanil pharmacokinetics in obese versus lean patients. Anesthesiology. 1998 Sep;89(3): 562-573.

[32] Ogunnaike BO, Jones SB, Jones DB, Provost D, Whitten CW. Anesthetic considerations for bariatric surgery. Anesth Analg. 2002 Dec;95(6):1793-1805.

[33] Perilli V, Sollazzi L, Bozza P, Modesti C, Chierichini A, Tacchino RM, Ranieri R. The effects of the reverse trendelenburg position on respiratory mechanics and blood gases in morbidly obese patients during bariatric surgery. Anesth Analg. 2000 Dec;91(6): 1520-1525.

[34] Remístico PP, Araújo S, de Figueiredo LC, Aquim EE, Gomes LM, Sombrio ML, Ambiel SD. Impact of alveolar recruitment maneuver in the postoperative period of videolaparoscopic bariatric surgery. Rev Bras Anestesiol. 2011 Mar-Apr;61(2):163-8, 169-76, 88-94.

[35] Talab HF, Zabani IA, Abdelrahman HS, Bukhari WL, Mamoun I, Ashour MA, Sadeq BB, El Sayed SI. Intraoperative ventilatory strategies for prevention of pulmonary atelectasis in obese patients undergoing laparoscopic bariatric surgery. Anesth Analg. 2009 Nov;109(5): 1511-1516.

[36] Valenza F, Vagginelli F, Tiby A, Francesconi S, Ronzoni G, Guglielmi M, Zappa M, Lattuada E, Gattinoni L. Effects of the beach chair position, positive end-expiratory pressure, and pneumoperitoneum on respiratory function in morbidly obese patients during anesthesia and paralysis. Anesthesiology. 2007 Nov;107(5): 725-732.

[37] Pelosi P, Gregoretti C. Perioperative management of obese patients. Best Pract Res Clin Anaesthesiol. 2010 Jun;24(2): 211-225.

[38] Kehlet H. Multimodal approach to control postoperative pathophysiology and rehabilitation. *Br J Anaesth* 1997;78:606-617.

[39] Wind J, Polle SW, Fung Kon Jin PH, et al. Systematic review of enhanced recovery programmes in colonic surgery. *Br J Surg* 2006;93:800-809.

[40] Varandhan, K.K., Neal K.R., Dejong C.H.C., Fearon K.C.H., Ljunqqvist O., Lobo D.N. et al. The enhanced recovery after surgery (ERAS) pathway for patients undergoing major elective open colorectal surgery: a meta-analysis of randomized trials. Clin. Nutr 2010, Aug;29(4):434-440.

[41] Van Bree S, Vlug M, Bemelman W, et. al. Faster recovery of gastrointestinal transit after laparoscopy and fast-track care in patients undergoing colonic surgery. Gastroenterology 2011;141:872-880.

[42] Lobo D.N., Bostock K.A., Neal K.R., et al. Effect of salt and water balance on recovery of gastrointestinal function after elective colonic resection: a randomised controlled trial. Lancet 2002; 359: 1812-1818.

[43] Kehlet. H. Multimodal approach to postoperative recovery.Curr Opin Crit Care 2009, 15: 355–358.

Chapter 3

Abdominal Surgery: Advances in the Use of Ultrasound-Guided Truncal Blocks for Perioperative Pain Management

Jens Børglum and Kenneth Jensen

Additional information is available at the end of the chapter

http://dx.doi.org/10.5772/48255

1. Introduction

1.1. Anatomical considerations

In the order to get an overview of the mechanisms for the conduction of pain stimulus from the abdominal area it is clearly important to refresh the memory concerning some of the basic anatomical considerations. This knowledge constitutes an important factor with the on-going quest of providing efficient and safe post- and perioperative pain management to patients undergoing abdominal surgery.

1.2. Visceral innervation

The viscera are innervated by the vagal nerve (parasympathetic innervation) and by the splanchnic nerves (sympathetic innervation). The splanchnic nerves carry both visceral efferent and afferent nerve fibers. The sensory (or afferent) part of the splanchnic nerves reach the spinal column at certain spinal segments. Table 1 attempts to give a brief overview of the visceral innervation by the sympathetic autonomic system.

If post- or perioperative pain sensations are predominantly transmitted via the autonomic nervous system, then the choice of analgesic management would today primarily rely on continuous intrathecal and especially epidural infusions of local anaesthetic. It is also possible to block central visceral pain conduction with thoracic paravertebral blockade or maybe even with the novel quadratus lumborum block (Carney 2011) We will deal with these blocks later in this chapter. Finally, opioids administered either orally or intravenously will also reduce visceral pain significantly.

Greater splanchnic nerve	Th5-Th9(10)	Celiac ganglia
Lesser splanchnic nerve	Th10-Th11	Superior mesenteric & Aorticorenal ganglia
Least splanchnic nerve	Th10	Renal plexus
Lumbar splanchnic nerves	L1-L2	Inferior mesenteric ganglia & ganglia of intermesenteric and hypogastric plexuses
Sacral splanchnic nervers	Sacral part of sympathetic trunk	Inferior hypogastric plexus and ganglia to the pelvic vicera

Table 1. Visceral innervation by the sympathetic autonomic system

1.3. Innervation of the anterolateral abdominal wall by the thoracolumbar spinal nerves

The innervation of the anterolateral abdominal wall by the somatic nervous system arises from the anterior rami of the thoracolumbar spinal nerves (Th6-L1) (Børglum 2011). Branches from the anterior rami include the intercostal nerves (Th6-T11), the subcostal nerve (Th12), and the iliohypogastric and ilioinguinal nerves (L1). Furthermore, Th6-Th12 nerves provide motor innervation to the pyramidalis and rectus muscles in the anterior abdomen, and Th6-L1 nerves innervate the intercostal muscles, the external and internal oblique muscles, the transversus abdominis muscles and also provide sensory innervation to the parietal peritoneum (Børglum 2011). However, many previous descriptions of the thoracolumbar spinal nerves innervating the abdominal wall have been inconsistent leading to misunderstanding and faulty attempts to provide sufficient anaesthesia (Rozen 2008). Conducting a thorough cadaveric study including comprehensive tracing of nerves and their branches Rozen et al. were able to describe the pattern and course of all thoracolumbar nerves innervating the anterior abdominal wall. The thoracolumbar nerves were found to travel as multiple mixed segmental nerves (running with their accompanying blood vessels), which branch and communicate widely within the neurovascular plane called the transversus abdominis plane (TAP) (Rozen 2008). Such large branch communications were found antero-laterally (the intercostal plexus – Th6-Th9), and in plexuses that run with the deep circumflex iliac artery (DCIA) (the classical TAP plexus – Th10-L1) and the deep inferior epigastric artery (DIEA) (rectus sheath plexus – Th6-L1) (Børglum 2012, Rozen 2008). Segmental nerves Th6 to Th9 emerged from the costal margin to enter the TAP between the midline and the anterior axillary line. Th6 entered the TAP just lateral to the linea alba, while Th7-Th9 emerged from the costal margin at increasingly lateral positions. It was also found that Th9 emerged from the costal margin either medial (predominantly) or lateral to the anterior axillary line (Rozen 2008).

2. Truncal blocks

2.1. History

Dr. Louis Gaston Labat was a pioneer in the world of regional anaesthesia. In the early 20th century, he brought to the United States knowledge he had acquired from his mentor, the

French surgery professor Victor Pauchet. Thus, the spread of regional anaesthesia in the United States was greatly facilitated by the work of Dr. Gaston Labat. Recruited to work at the Mayo Clinic, Dr. Labat there published his original textbook, *Regional Anesthesia,* in which he laid out his techniques to the next generation of physician specialists (Labat 1922, Bacon 2002). Regional anaesthesia in the United States was popularized by Dr. Labat's book, and many physician anaesthesiologists in the 1920s and 1930s learned regional techniques this way. Most interestingly concerning the current chapter, in relation to abdominal operations, regional anaesthesia had already then been found to provide superior muscle relaxation with fewer complications than deep ether anaesthesia. Dr. Labat has also been given credit for the posterior approach to splanchnic nerve block,use of intercostal block instead of paravertebral block for breast surgery, the use of abdominal field blocks, level of dural puncture and many other regional anaesthetic techniques (Côté 2003). Further, in the early 1920s Dr. Labat wrote about the combined caudal, trans-sacral and paravertebral (lower lumbar) block for resection of the rectum. He also elaborated extensively on other regional techniques: "With the abdominal field block procedure, colostomy is performed painlessly, provided the patient is not too obese and the mesocolon is not too short. Exploration is possible in the majority of cases, if gentleness is used. The sacral block, consisting of the caudal or epidural and transsacral block, added to the paravertebral block of the last three lumbar nerves on both sides, constitutes the method of choice for the posterior resection of the carcinomatous rectum and rectosigmoid". Thus, this very brief historical entry highlights the fact that the use of truncal blocks certainly is not a new phenomenon in anaesthesia practice. The old masters relied on landmark-based techniques as well as a thorough understanding of anatomy and anatomical variations.

2.2. Evidence-based medicine

In 2010 Abrahams et al. performed a systematic search of the medical literature in the quest to describe evidence-based medicine in relation to ultrasound (US) guidance for truncal block administration (Abrahams 2010). In this review article it is mentioned that anaesthesia and analgesia of the trunk can be achieved with perineural injections, which could have several advantages compared with neuraxial blockade; i.e. reduced sympathectomy, less severe consequences of infection or bleeding at the injection site, minimal interference with bladder and bowel function, and less incidence of lower extremity motor weakness (Abrahams 2010). It is also clearly stated that Thoracic Paravertebral blocks (TPVB) from Th6-L1, TAP blocks, Rectus Sheath (RS) blocks, and Ilioinguinal and Iliohypogastric nerve (IIN and IHN) blocks can provide anaesthesia and analgesia of the abdominal wall. Abraham et al. did not compare the efficacy of various truncal blocks against each other or against the golden standard of the continuous epidural blockade. In the following we will go through the most common truncal blocks suitable for the purpose of alleviating the patients from pain following abdominal surgery. Table 2 provides an overview of the recommended ultrasound-guided (USG) truncal nerve blocks specifically in relation to abdominal surgical procedures.

Truncal nerve blockade	Indications
Bilateral Dual – Transversus Abdominal Plane (BD-TAP) block	Fig. 1: Intercostal TAP block (IC-TAP) block providing anaesthesia to the upper abdomen (Th6-Th9) (PPM) Fig. 2: Classical TAP block (CL-TAP) providing anaesthesia to the lower abdomen (Th10-Th12) (PPM)
Ilioinguinal/iliohypogastric nerve (IIN/IHN) block (L1)	Fig. 3: Open and laparoscopic inguinal hernia repair (PPM)
Rectus sheath (RS) block (Th6-L1)	Fig. 4: Midline incisions and trochar holes (PPM)
Intercostal nerve (ICN) block (single or multiple injection technique)	Fig.5: Cholecystectomy, trochar holes high in the epigastric area (PPM)
Thoracic paravertebral block (TPVB)	Fig. 6: Providing anaesthesia both to the upper (Th6-Th9) and lower (Th10-L1) abdomen depending on the site of administration and the volume of local anaesthetic. Has the potential to block the visceral pain in addition to the somatic sensory pain.
Quadratus lumborum (QL) block	Fig. 7: Seems to be able to provide anaesthesia from the Th5 to the L1. Is currently still rather inadequately described. Seems to have the potential to block the visceral pain in addition to the somatic sensory pain.

Table 2. Overview of recommended truncal nerve blocks specifically in relation to abdominal surgical procedures. Indications only include postoperative pain management (PPM).

2.3. Education in ultrasound-guided (USG) peripheral nerve blocks

In order to enhance the clinical implementation process, to support further education and to advance improvements in clinical practice, the American Society of Regional Anesthesia and Pain Medicine (ASRA) and the European Society of Regional Anaesthesia and Pain Therapy (ESRA) encouraged all institutions that conduct USG PNB to support a quality improvement process (Sites 2010). The joint committee of ASRA and ESRA advocated a focus on the following issues: (i) ten common tasks used when performing an ultrasound-guided nerve block, (ii) the core competencies and skills associated with UGS PNB, and (iii) a training practice pathway for postgraduate anaesthesiologists and a residency-based training pathway (Sites 2010). Table 3 lists the first proposal from the joint committee of ASRA and ESRA.

High block expertise requires both anatomical knowledge and extensive hands-on experience (Jensen 2011, Orebaugh 2009). In this pursuit it is probably wise to adhere to the principles or EFSUMB (www.efsumb.org) when dividing practitioners into various catagories (levels of expertice) when formulating a strategy for enhancing the continuous education of physicians. As to the other proposals regarding core competencies and skills associated with USG peripheral nerve blocks and the proposed training practice pathway at any institution, this chapter refers to the original publication (Sites 2010). Our primary aim with this chapter is to provide the reader with an easy pathway to perform USG truncal nerve blocks in daily clinical practise. The USG truncal nerve blocks can in reality be performed by any *trained* physician qualified in the field of emergency medicine, acute pain management and trauma as well as anaesthesiologists providing for surgical anaesthesia and postoperative pain management. In the following we will provide recommendations on how to perform the various USG truncal blocks and show relevant clinical photographs together with ultrasound recordings to advice the reader accordingly. However, it is necessary to mention early on, that the special field of USG truncal blocks differs from the performance of USG peripheral nerve blocks on the upper and lower extremities; i.e. with USG truncal blocks you very rarely actually see the nerves ultrasonographically. Rather, the focus for the physician must be on the surrounding perineural structures (muscle layer, fascia, neurovascular plane, bone etc.) and a thorough knowledge of anatomy.

1	Visualize key landmark structures including blood vessels, muscles, fascia, and bone
2	Identify the nerves or plexus on short-axis imaging
3	Confirm normal anatomy and recognize anatomic variation(s)
4	Plan for a needle approach that avoids unnecessary tissue trauma
5	Maintain an aseptic technique with respect to the ultrasound equipment
6	Follow the needle under real-time visualization as it advances toward the target
7	Consider a secondary confirmation technique, such as nerve stimulation
8	When the needle tip is presumed to be in the correct position, inject a small volume of a test solution. If solution is not visualized during this test injection, presume that the needle tip is intravascular or out of the imaging plane.
9	Make necessary needle adjustments if an undesired pattern of local anaesthetic spread is visualized. The visualization of local anaesthetic should occur through the entirety of the injection to avoid an intravascular injection
10	Maintain traditional safety guidelines including the presence of resuscitation equipment, frequent aspiration, intravascular test dosing, standard monitoring, patient response, and assessment of injection characteristics

Table 3. Ten tasks helpful in performing USG peripheral nerve blocks. (Sites 2012)

2.4. Transversus abdominis plane (TAP) block

The idea of the TAP block is to anaesthetize part of - or the entire - abdominal wall instead of using intrathecal or epidural techniques, that may or may not elicit more negative side effects by the application. By adhering to this principle one would block the nerves as peripheral as possible but only as centrally a necessary (to quote Professor Peter Marhofer, Austria). The technique builds on anaesthetizing the peripheral nerves to the abdomen using a direct approach. Since the first description of the TAP block technique by Rafi (or something very similar to what it is conceived as today), this block has been increasingly used to provide somatic anaesthesia of the antero-lateral abdominal wall (Rafi 2001, Abrahams 2010, Petersen 2010, Børglum 2011, Koscielniak-Nielsen 2011, Børglum 2012). This landmark-based blind approach to deposit local anaesthetic at the neurovascular plane was since thoroughly described by McDonnell et al. and further documented using computerized tomography (McDonnell 2004, 2007). As of today, it would seem that four different TAP block approaches are in common use. First, let us begin with the landmark-based blind approach at the triangle of Petit. McDonnell et al. and Carney et al. have provided ample evidence with many scientific publications for the huge success when using their TAP block approach where ultrasound guidance is not used (McDonnell 2007, Carney 2009, 2011), but where extensive dermatomal anaesthesia is achived and postoperatively pain management is improved significantly for a great many surgical procedures. Second, we find the USG approach to the TAP very well described by El-Dawlatly et al. and Shibata et al. Both use two separate injections deposited at the lateral classical TAP plexus; i.e. one injection on each hemi-abdomen (above the iliac crest and below the thoracic cage) (El-Dawlatly 2009, Shibata 2007). This simple and very efficient technique is probably the method most commonly used today. Thirdly, we find the brilliant classification by Hebbard et al. where the USG continuous oblique subcostal transversus abdominis plane blockade technique is described (Hebbard 2010). Dr. Hebbard must be thankfully accredited to address the issue of providing consistent anaesthesia to both the lower (Th10-L1) and upper (Th6-Th9) abdominal wall on a continuous basis. In addition, Dr. Hebbard´s research has showed that it possible to use more peripheral approaches to continuous block the entire abdominal wall. Dr. Hebbard has however clearly expressed that his technique for providing safe and continuous anaesthesia to the entire abdomen requires considerable skills and serious anatomical knowledge (Hebbard 2010). Having said that, one must not rule out that McDonnell et al. have also found their landmarked-based and blind approach to be able to anaesthetize the entire abdominal wall for an extended period. Finally – and fourth – is our own approach called the bilateral dual TAP (BD-TAP) block based on four single shot injections with the aim to provide anaesthesia to the entire abdominal wall in a fast and safe sequence (Børglum 2011, Børglum 2012). Our method does not rely on relatively lengthy or sophisticated methods for the insertion of catheters; rather our technique relies on simple anatomical knowledge and structured ultrasonographic recognition (Børglum 2011, Børglum 2012). The BD-TAP block will normally take the well-trained anaesthesiologist approximately 5-6 minutes to perform. Probably even shorter time if the block is administered prior to surgery. The BD-TAP block will anaesthetize the dermatomes Th6-Th12, the antero-medial muscles of the abdominal wall and the underlying parietal peritoneum. It would also be fair to say that the BD-TAP block builds to some extent on a "mixture" of previously described techniques by El-Dawlatly et al. and Shibata et al. as well as Dr. Hebbards research (El-Dawlatly 2009, Shibata 2007, Hebbard 2010). In addition, the BD-TAP technique has been proved *not* to result in inhibition of the accessory respiratory function attributed to the abdominal wall muscles – mainly forced expiration (Petersen 2011). The efficacy of the BD-TAP block technique has been ascertained by magnetic resonance imaging (MRI) (Børglum 2012), and it seems obvious that it is not possible to anaesthetize the entire abdominal wall (TH6-L1) with the so-called lateral classical TAP block technique alone, but that the intercostal TAP plexus in the upper abdomen (epigastric area) must also be anaesthetized by a direct approach in addition.

Generally speaking when considering outcome measures of the various techniques, TAP blocks have been described as an effective component of multimodal postoperative analgesic protocols for a wide variety of abdominal surgical procedures including laparotomy for colorectal surgery, open and laparoscopic appendectomy, caesarean section, abdominal hysterectomy, laparoscopic cholecystectomy, open prostatectomy and renal transplant surgery. In an uncontrolled study, patients undergoing lower abdominal gynaecological surgery received bilateral TAP block catheters, and the authors found an average pain at rest and on movement below 2 on a 10-point VAS scale for up to 48 hours postoperatively, with no occurrences of nausea or side effects (Fujita 2012). Compared to systemic opioids, patients receiving TAP blocks after major abdominal surgery had less pain up to 24 hours postoperatively than non-TAP block groups, but in that study no statistical differences were found with respect to nausea (Siddiqui 2011). The benefits of TAP blocks are so far measured in relation to reduced postoperative opioid requirements, lower pain scores or a reduction in opioid-related side effects (Shin 2011). As an example, a meta-analysis of 7 studies demonstrated an average reduction in 24-hour morphine consumption of 22 mg compared with systemic opioids, and TAP blocks were associated with reduced early postoperative pain VAS in 4 of the 7 studies (Petersen 2010). Postoperative sedation, as well as PONV, was marginally reduced in patients having TAP blocks administered. Newer studies confirm these findings, and also observe a higher patient satisfaction in the TAP block groups (Hivelin 2011). Despite the numerous descriptive studies on TAP blocks, however, results of comparative studies have been inconsistent. The current scientific evidence is lacking to definitively identify the surgical procedures, dosing, techniques, and timing that provide optimal analgesia following TAP block (Abdallah 2012).

2.4.1. Detailed description of the BD-TAP block

With the aim to render the entire abdominal wall pain-free after surgery (or during the surgical procedure) one must anaesthetize all the antero-lateral rami of the thoracoabdominal nerves (Th6-Th12). In doing so, one must anaesthetize both the intercostal TAP plexus (Th6-Th9) situated in the epigastric area just below the xiphoid process medially to the costal curvature (Fig. 1), and one must also target the lateral classical TAP plexus (Th10-Th12) situated in the lower abdomen. This must be done on both hemi-abdomens. When administering local anaesthetic to the uppermost branches of the intercostal TAP plexus the physician must use the USG intercostal TAP (IC-TAP) block, where the IC-TAP plexus lies in the fascial plane between the rectus abdominis (RA) muscle (or rather deep to the posterior rectus sheath) and the transversus abdominis (TA) muscle (Fig. 1). When blocking the lateral classical TAP (CL-TAP) plexus the point of skin penetration must be in the anterior axillary line above the iliac crest and below the thoracic cage (Fig. 2). The needle is then advanced posterior and increasingly lateral, and the point of injection will be in the middle axillary line between the internal oblique (IO) and TA muscles. Thus, the BD-TAP block technique can best be described as a fast and simple four-point USG single-shot TAP block approach. For all TAP blocks the patient is placed in a supine position, and a linear transducer (6-15 MHz) is placed with its medial end pointing medially (Fig. 1-2). The needle is inserted in-plane to the transducer in a medial to lateral direction with the endpoint in the fascial neurovascular plane between the RA and TA (IC-TAP block) or between the IO and TA (CL-TAP block). The spread of the injectate should be observed to be distributed within the neurovascular plane.

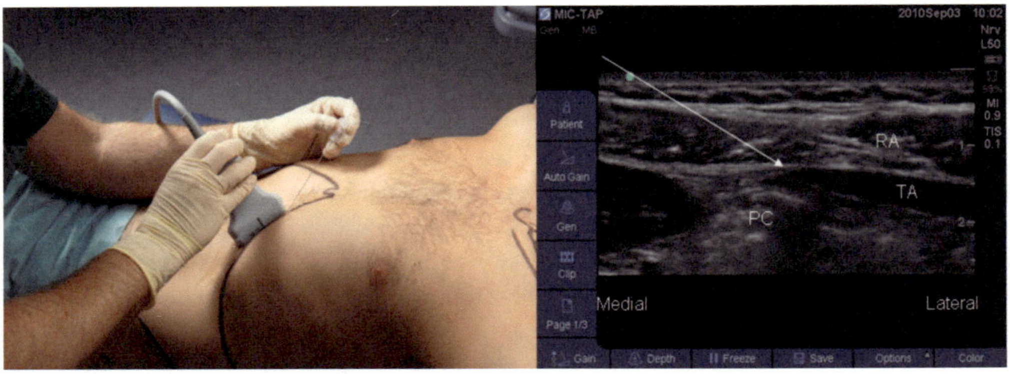

Figure 1. USG IC-TAP block (Th6-Th9). PC: peritoneal cavity.

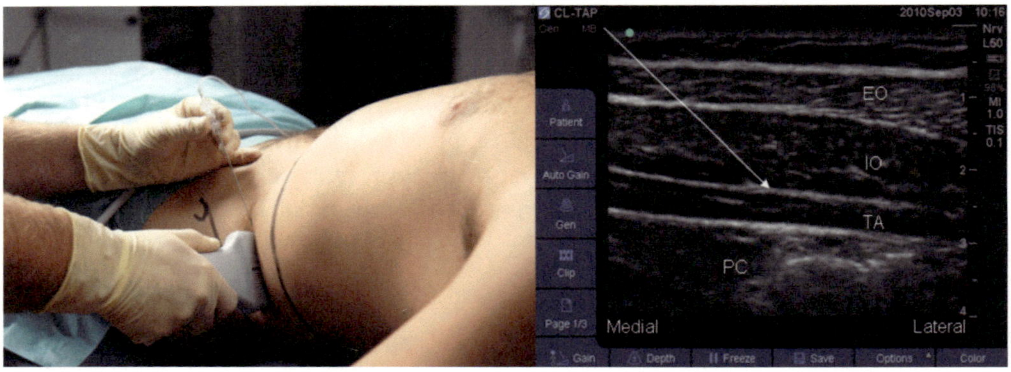

Figure 2. USG CL-TAP block (Th10-Th12). EO: external oblique muscle, PC: peritoneal cavity.

2.4.2. TAP block – A systematic review

Very recently a thorough systematic review concerning the various TAP blocks was published, and the review centres on postoperative analgesia following abdominal surgery (Abdallah et al. 2012). According to this systematic review improved analgesia was found in patients subjected to laparotomy for colorectal surgery, laparoscopic cholecystectomy, and open and laparoscopic appendectomy (Abdallah et al. 2012). Superior analgesic outcomes was also found when 15 mL of local anaesthetic or more was used per side, compared with lesser volumes, and TAP blocks performed in the triangle of Petit and along the midaxillary line both demonstrated some analgesic advantages (Abdallah et al. 2012). Finally, this systematic review also found that although the majority of trials reviewed suggested superior early pain control, they were unable to definitively identify the surgical procedures, local anaesthetic doses, techniques, and timing (pre- or post-incisional) that would ensure optimal analgesia following the TAP blocks. Thus, there is still much work to be done.

2.5. USG ilioinguinal/iliohypogastric nerve (IIN/IHN) block

This is a selective block of the ventral ramus of the L1. The IIN provides sensation to the upper medial part of the thigh and the upper part of the genitalia. The IHN provides sensation to the buttock and abdominal wall above the pubis (Abrahams 2010). In our own previous studies, we have been unable to register effective dermatomal anaesthesia of the L1 branch with our BD-TAP block technique, but other studies have shown the L1 branches to be blocked by other versions of the TAP block technique (Børglum 2012, Carney 2011). For the selective USG IIN/IHN block the patient is placed in a supine position, and the anterior superior iliac spine (ASIS) is localized by palpation first and since ultrasonographically (Fig. 3). A linear transducer (6-15 MHz) is placed with its lateral end at or just superior to the ASIS. The needle is inserted in-plane to the transducer in a lateral to medial direction, and the neurovascular plane between the IO and the TA is located. The IIN and IHN can often be seen together with the deep circumflex iliac artery in the neurovascular plane. This is rather specific for this particular truncal block, because trunk nerves are not as easily discovered by US as are the peripheral nerves of the upper and lower extremities. The tip of the needle is placed in this plane, and the spread of the injectate should be observed to expand in the fascial neurovascular plane (3).

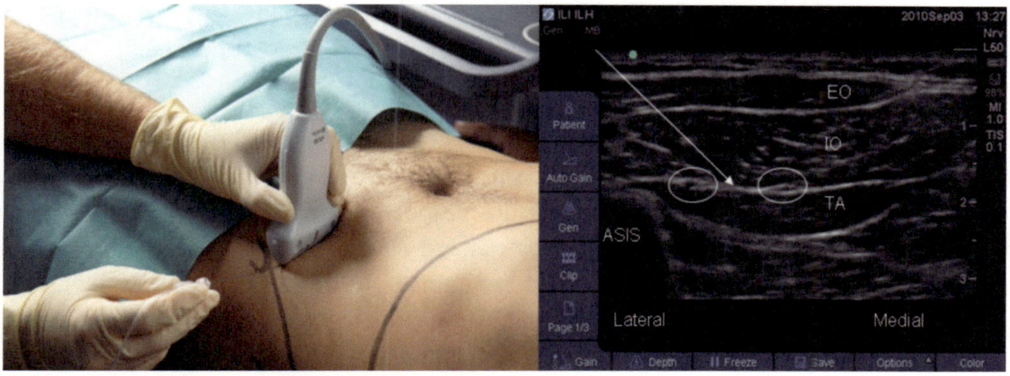

Figure 3. USG IIN/IHN block. EO: external oblique muscle.

Traditional techniques were landmark-based and relied on one or two facial "clicks", but the old techniques are largely abandoned now, since US imaging subsequent to the so-called blind blocks has demonstrated incorrect placement of the local anaesthetic administered (Weintraud 2008). The US technique is very well established already (Willschke 2005, Willschke 2006, Eichenberger 2007). Most IIN/IHN blocks are placed for analgesia after inguinal hernia repairs in children, but have also been shown to provide similar analgesia to caudal blocks during orchidopexy and hydrocele repair (Abrahams 2010). In his review article Dr. Abrahams gave the use of US guidance for the IIN/IHN block a Grade A recommendation (Abrahams 2010). Our own very recent study concerning primary open inguinal hernia repair (ad modum Lichtenstein) in adult males showed significant reduction in pain scores at mobilization and at rest in the group of patients having active bupivacaine USG IIN/IHN blocks administered prior to surgery (Bærentzen 2012). The pain scores were recorded when the patients arrived at the post anaesthesia care unit (PACU) and after 30 minutes stay. Pain at rest was similarly reduced in the active group at the time of discharge. Most importantly, patients with severe (NRS>5) and moderate (NRS>3) pain at mobilization and rest, respectively, were significantly reduced in the group of patients having the block (Bærentzen 2012). Thus, it would seem that the USG IIN/IHN block also has a place in the post- and perioperative pain management in adult patients.

2.6. USG rectus sheath (RS) block

The central portion of the anterior abdominal wall is innervated by the ventral branches of the thoracolumbar nerves (Th6-L1), and in the beginning of this chapter we have already mentioned the rectus sheath plexus and its anatomical position. The ventral branches lie deep to the RA muscle but ventral to the posterior rectus sheath. Since the tendinous inscriptions of the rectus muscle are not attached to the posterior RS the local anaesthetic administered into the spatial space can in theory spread both in the cranial and caudal direction. However, the RS block may have been over-shadowed by the various TAP block techniques, but the evidence base for its use is very good; i.e. a grade A recommendation for the use of US guidance for the RS block has been granted (Abrahams 2010). The RS block has been utilized to provide analgesia for midline incisions and laparoscopic procedures (Ferguson 1996, Abrahams 2010). RS blocks may also be effective in reducing postoperative pain in upper abdominal surgery as an alternative method to epidural analgesia in anti-coagulated patients (Osaka 2010).

However, we find that the RS block has a potential drawback, since the risk for inadvertent injections deep to the posterior RS (intra-peritoneal) seems to be higher that for the USG TAP blocks where the TA muscle lies deep to the point of injection (Dolan 2009). To our knowledge, no comparison between TAP blocks and RS blocks has yet been done. For the selective USG RS block, the patient is placed in a supine position, and a linear transducer (6-15 MHz) is placed with its medial end just above the linea alba (LA) (Fig. 4). The needle is inserted in-plane to the transducer in a medial to lateral direction, and the division between the belly of the rectus abdominis muscle and the posterior rectus sheath is visualized. The tip of the needle is placed in this space. The spread of the injectate should be observed to advance in a lateral direction.

2.7. USG intercostal nerve (ICN) block: Parasagittal plane

The thoracoabdominal nerves Th6-Th11 are all intercostal nerves *per se*, before they become abdominal nerves when they leave the thoracic cage and contribute to the formation of the

IC-TAP, CL-TAP and RS-TAP plexuses in the anterolateral abdominal wall (Rozen 2008). Thus the potential to provide efficient abdominal analgesia employing US guidance to block the intercostal nerves are obviously there if a multiple injection technique is used. In the past, the landmark-based (blind) technique has been employed to provide analgesia for various surgical procedures in the abdominal area; i.e. following renal transplantation, cholecystectomy and appendectomy (Knowles 1998, Vieira 2003, Bunting 1988). It would seem to be obvious that the USG ICN block (multiple injection technique) could very well be used postoperatively; i.e. either as an effective rescue block or because TAP blocks were not possible due to surgical incisions, tissue swelling etc. For the selective USG ICN block the patient is placed in the lateral decubitus position, and a linear transducer (6-15 MHz) is placed in a sagittal paravertebral plane (Fig. 5). The needle is inserted in-plane to the transducer in a cranial to caudal direction, and the three intercostal muscles (external, internal and innermost) are visualized between two costae. The tip of the needle is placed in the fascial plane between the internal and innermost intercostal muscles. The spread of the injectate should be observed to occur in this fascial plane. It is very important to visualize the tip of the needle at all times and its close proximity to the parietal pleura.

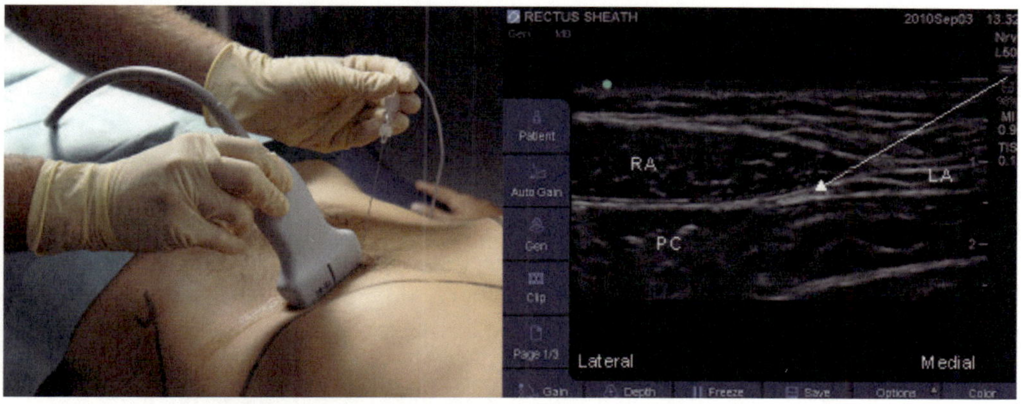

Figure 4. USG RS block. PC: peritoneal cavity, LA: linia alba.

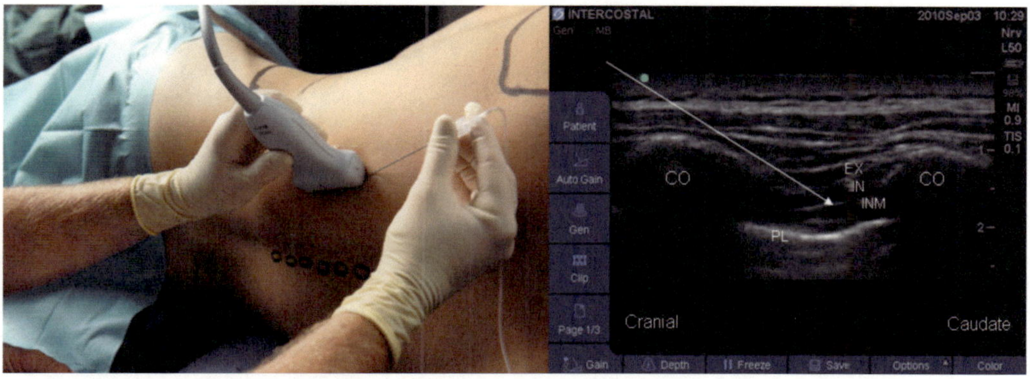

Figure 5. USG ICN block: parasagittal plane. CO: costa, EX,IN,INM: external, internal, innermost intercostal muscles, PL: pleura.

2.8. USG Thoracic Paravertebral block (TPVB)

The conventional technique of a TPVB involves inserting the needle perpendicular to all planes, making contact with the transverse process, and then walking off the bone with the needle until the physician feels the loss of resistance when penetrating deep to the internal intercostal membrane and entering the thoracic paravertebral space (TPVS). The TPVB has been used to provide pain relief for many surgical procedures in the abdominal area (Naja 2002, Moussa 2008, Ho 2004, Berta 2008). Conducting an USG TPVB or using the traditional landmark-based methods is the technique of injecting local anaesthetic adjacent to the thoracic vertebra close to the actual site where spinal nerves emerge from the intervertebral foramina. This results in ipsi-lateral somatic and sympathetic nerve blockade in multiple contiguous thoracic dermatomes above and below the site of injection (Karmakar 2001). How much dermatomal anaesthesia in the abdominal area results from specific volumes of local anaesthetic is to our knowledge still not fully elucidated, at least when it concerns the USG TPVBs. There is bound to be considerable individual variations as well. From previous studies it would seem that the point of injection within the TPVS must influence the distribution pattern of a paravertebral blockade. Apparently, injections made in the more ventral part of the TPVS, supposedly anterior to the endothoracic fascia, will result in a multisegmental longitudinal spreading pattern (evaluated by radiographic spreading patterns), whereas injections dorsal to the endothoracic fascia will result in a cloud-like spreading pattern, with only limited distribution over adjacent segments (Naja 2004). Whether US guidance can make the administration of local anaesthetic more beneficial remains to be evaluated in future studies. Even when using the USG technique, the endothoracic fascia is very difficult to visualize if at all possible with the current ultrasound machines. The TPVB is effective in treating pain of resulting from surgery in the chest and abdomen (Karmakar 2001). The potential advantage over the various TAP blocks could be that the visceral pain is more reliably blocked with the TPVB. Further, the potential failure rates and complications using the traditional techniques have already been brilliantly described previously (Lönnqvist 1995). Finally, insertion of catheters using the USG technique in the TPVS is indeed possible with at high success rate, thus making this technique a potential replacement of the epidural continuous infusion catheters (Renes 2010).

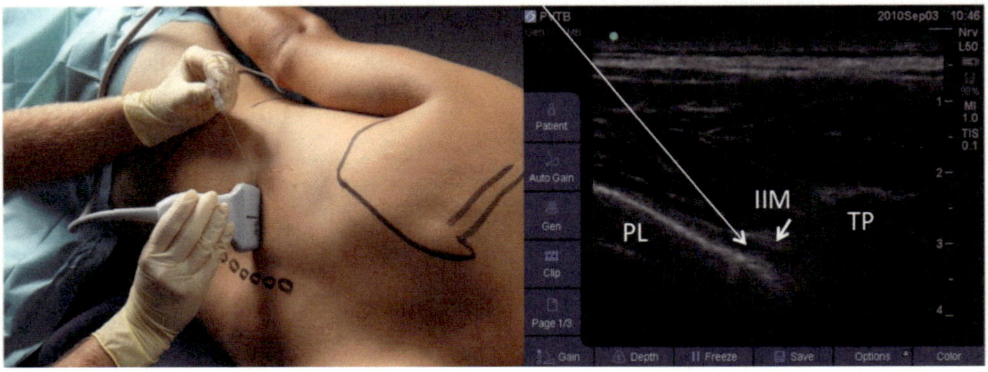

Figure 6. USG TPVB block. IIM: Internal intercostal membrane (continuous with the superior costotransverse ligament medially), PL: Pleura, TP: Transverse process

For the selective USG TPVB block the patient is placed in the lateral decubitus position, and a linear transducer (6-15 MHz) is placed parallel to and in-between two costae in an axial transverse plane (Fig. 6). It is important to visualize the pleura very clearly at all times. The transducer is then gradually aligned in a medial direction until the acoustic shadow of the transverse process is clearly visualized in the medial part of the sonographic image. The needle is inserted in-plane to the transducer in a lateral to medial direction until the tip of the needle is seen to penetrate the internal intercostal membrane. We do not recommend that the needle tip should be advanced under the acoustic shadow of the transverse process. Rather, we recommend that the spread of the injectate should be observed to occur above the pleura in the triangular space (which is the TPVS) and thus depressing the pleura and filling up the TPVS. It is very important to visualize the tip of the needle at all times and its close proximity to the parietal pleura.

2.9. USG Quadratus Lumborum (QL) block – the "new kid on the block"

As we are approaching the end of the description of the various USG truncal blocks we would like to introduce the reader to the "new kid on the block". The so-called Blanco block (as it is known by some anaesthetists in the United Kingdom) is an USG block administered to the quadratus lumborum space first described by Professor R. Blanco in May 2007 during his presentation at ESRA 2007 at the XXVI Annual ESRA Congress in Valencia, Spain. Professor Blanco describes a potential space posterior to the abdominal wall muscles and lateral to the quadratus lumborum muscle. Thus, this new block has also been called the Quadratus lumborum (QL) block. It has been used in abdominoplasties, caesarean sections and lower abdominal operations since 2006 providing complete pain relief in the distribution area from Th6 to L1 dermatomes. Apparently, in operations with peritoneal involvement the morphine consumption was significantly reduced to less than 30% of the control groups. It is hard however, to find any solid scientific evidence to support these findings in the literature, and much of the knowledge of the QL block relies regrettably to this day on personal communication, which is certainly not the best of documentation. Much research effort at many centres is currently directed towards the description and qualification of this new block, and we have found it highly relevant to include the block in this chapter, since the block holds some very positive potential benefits. If may well be seen as a lumbar approach to the TPVS. The block apparently produces distribution of the local anaesthetic extending proximally and over both sides of the surface of the QL muscle, in between the anterior and intermediate layers of the thoracolumbar fascias It also pushes the fascia transversalis and the perinephric fat towards the peritoneum without the risk of intrabdominal puncture. The block does not rely on the feeling of any pops or fascial clicks because depending of the angle of the needle several pops can be felt without reaching the target zone, which is lateral to the quadratus lumborum muscle. Actually, the block has never been intended to be conducted without the use of US guidance, and the block is thus a purely USG block. In an absolutely brilliant paper by Carney et al. the block is compared to other TAP block techniques using volunteers rather than patients (Carney 2011). Dr. Carney found that there was a non-contiguous paravertebral, epidural and lymphatic contrast enhancement Th5-Th10 in one subject, and similarly contrast at Th6-Th10 in two other subjects (Carney 2011).

Carney et al. concluded that the posterior USG approach (as they have named the QL block in their recent publication) produced a more extensive, predictable and posterior spread of contrast, similar to that seen with their own landmark-based and blind approach at the triangle of Petit. The contrast extended postero-medially to the paravertebral region from the 5th thoracic vertebral level rostrally, to the first lumbar vertebral level caudally, indicating that this US guidance approach is the optimal site for injection to reproduce the analgesia of the blind landmark TAP block favoured by Dr. McDonnell and Dr. Carney. Fig. 7 depicts one method to administer the USG guided QL block as we have found it most easy to perform in our daily clinical practise (Jensen 2012). Again, the patient rests in a supine position. We have found it easier to conduct the block using a low frequency transducer (2-6 MHz) as compared to a linear transducer. The low frequency transducer is placed on the lateral abdomen above the iliac crest and below the thoracic cage. The transducer is then gradually aligned in a more posterior and lateral direction parallel to the inter-crista line. It is always possible to observe, that the TA muscle becomes aponeurotic, and this aponeurosis is followed until the QL muscle is clearly visualized. Thus, it is indeed possible to visualize the QL muscle lateral and posterior to the abdominal wall muscles. It is also clearly possible to visualize the thoracolumbar fascia at the lateral edge of the QL muscle. We have set this to be the point of injection of local anaesthetic. Following the injection we could observe the local anaesthetic spread along the ventral side of the QL muscle. Apparently this block results in a block that is longer lasting and more extensive than what we have previously observed with the BD-TAP block, but it remains to be further elucidated in RCT trials.

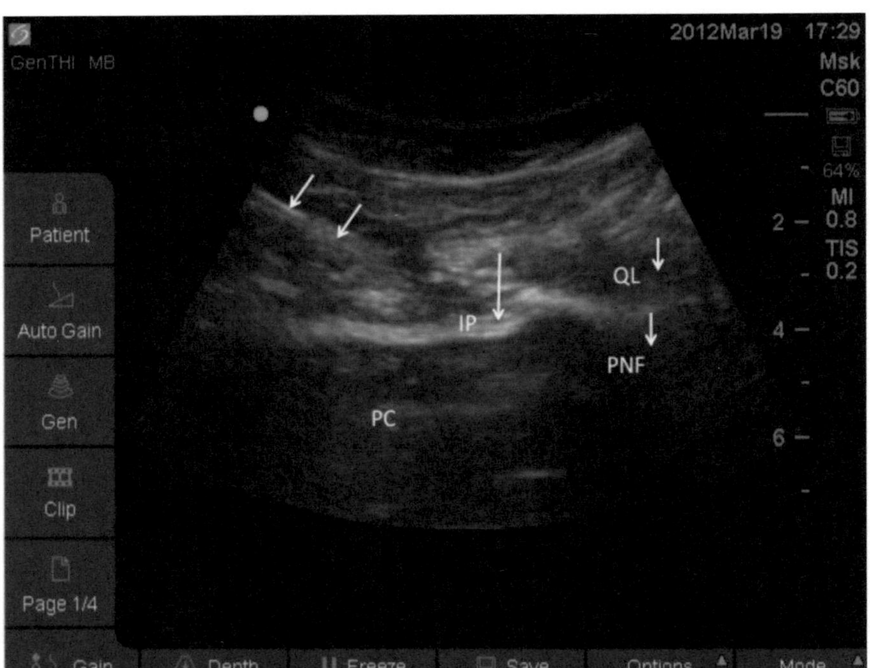

Figure 7. USG QL block. Arrows in upper left corner indicating needle shaft approaching in a medial to lateral-posterior direction towards the injection point (IP). PC: Peritoneal cavity, IP: Injection point, QL: Quadratus lumborum muscle, PNF: Perinephric fat.

3. Epidural analgesia

3.1. General physiology of the epidural

Epidural analgesia is an effective method of anaesthetizing the sensory nerves to the abdominal wall. The impulse conduction of sensory roots protruding from the spinal cord is considerably reduced in a dermatomal fashion, optimally extending from the 4th to the 12th thoracic dermatome. Not all spinothalamic nerve transmission is reduced however, and some sensory input is perceived by the brain (Lund 1991). An element of habituation (so-called tachyphylaxis) is also present, in which the nerve roots require increasing amounts of local anaesthetic to maintain a sufficient nerve block over days. This inconvenient effect may be reduced by the addition of opioids, administered epidurally or systemically. Common side effects include a subsidiary block of the sympathetic trunk in the dermatomes anaesthetized, causing arteriole relaxation, reduced peripheral vascular resistance with hypotension and reflex tachycardia; motor block of the lower extremities when the epidural extends below thoracic dermatomes; and central nervous system side effects such as drowsiness, nausea or pruritus when opioids or other drugs are added to the local anaesthetic. The placement of an epidural catheter requires some experience, and the handling of an epidural catheter is particularly resource heavy for infusion maintenance and monitoring of potential side effects.

3.2. The epidural catheter in a historical perspective

The benefits and risks of epidural analgesia have been extensively documented ever since its introduction almost 100 years ago (Thompson 1917). In the past ten years alone, more than two publications have appeared every single day on the subject, equally distributed between analgesic effects in major surgery, obstetric anaesthesia, side effects and technical aspects (Jensen 2012). Apart from subarachnoidal analgesia, which was first introduced in 1898 (Bier 1899), it is hard to imagine a method of analgesia having been similarly subjected to scientific study. In the case of spinal anaesthesia, the foundation for its use is still overwhelming by its significant reduction in perioperative morbidity and mortality compared to general anaesthesia (Rodgers 2000). Epidural analgesia is a well-established technique that is often regarded as the gold standard in postoperative pain management. However, newer and evidence-based outcome data show that its benefits are not as significant as previously believed, and that these benefits are probably limited to high-risk patients undergoing major abdominal surgery receiving epidural analgesia with local anaesthetic drugs only. There is increasing evidence that less invasive regional analgesic techniques are as effective as epidural analgesia, and while pain relief associated with epidurals can be outstanding, clinicians expect more from this invasive, high-cost, labour-intensive technique (Niraj 2009; Rawal 2012). A plethora of cardiovascular, neurologic and infectious side effects of epidural analgesia have been published, and given its modest success rate (at 70-80%) and the potential of motor block of the lower extremities, the scale is beginning to tip in the direction of USG truncal nerve blocks, in particular when the need for short-term analgesia of the abdominal wall is anticipated or when patients are not high-risk.

3.3. Physiological reactions to surgery

Invasive surgery induces a combination of local response to tissue injury and generalized activation of systemic metabolic and hormonal pathways via afferent nerve pathways and the central nervous system. The local inflammatory responses and the parallel neurohumoral pathways are linked through complex signalling networks. The magnitude of the response is related to the site of injury (greater in abdomen or thorax) and the extent of the trauma. The changes include alterations in metabolic, hormonal, inflammatory, and immune systems that collectively are termed the stress response. Integral to the stress response are the effects of nociceptive afferent stimuli on systemic and pulmonary vascular resistance, heart rate and blood pressure. Opioid doses required to provide analgesia are less than those required for haemodynamic stability in response to surgery, and these are in turn less than those required to suppress most aspects of the stress response. In contrast to this considerable dose dependency, neuraxial nerve blocks allow blockade of the afferent and efferent sympathetic pathways at relatively low doses resulting in profound suppression of hemodynamic and stress responses to surgery (Wolf 2012). Intraoperative stress may therefore suppress the adaptive immune system. Abolished pro-inflammatory lymphocyte function is associated with higher risk of infection and postoperative complications. During major abdominal surgery, plasma concentrations of epinephrine and cortisol are significantly lower in the epidural group compared to the non-epidural group. Lymphocyte numbers and T-helper cells are significantly higher in the epidural group on day one, whereas no significant differences may be detected among IL-2, HLA-DR, or the postoperative clinical course. Intraoperative use of a thoracic epidural catheter may therefore reduce stress response and prevent stress-induced perioperative impairment of pro-inflammatory lymphocyte function (Ahlers 2008). However, other studies find that epidural analgesia cannot suppress postoperative lymphocyte apoptosis, increases in cortisol, CRP or ESR compared with general anaesthesia, so the evidence is equivocal (Papadima 2009). Epidurals modify the electrical activity of the heart in addition to ventricular function and wall motion. Improvements in regional blood flow and a reduction of the major determinants of cardiac oxygen consumption lead to less severity of the ischemic injury. Although epidural analgesia negatively affects the performance of intercostal muscles, is spares diaphragmatic function and, when limited to the first five thoracic segments, affects pulmonary volumes to a lesser extent. Improved gastrointestinal blood flow and motility are clear in animals, and in clinical studies epidurals have been shown to improve recovery after major abdominal surgery. Liver perfusion increases with thoracic but not lumbar epidural analgesia after major abdominal surgery in most patients (Kortgen 2009). However, its use alone cannot prevent postoperative morbidity and mortality (Clemente 2008). Overall though, the evidence is strong that epidural analgesia is superior to systemic opioids after major abdominal surgery (www.postoppain.org). Postoperative pulmonary function, mobilization, food intake and general well-being are all increased (Catro-Alves 2011). Its benefit on postoperative analgesia is most evident in surgery involving high-risk surgery or high-risk patients (Siriussawakul 2010; van Lier 2011; Panaretou 2012).

3.4. Outcome studies with epidurals

Data generally indicate that the perioperative use of regional anaesthesia and analgesia may be associated with improvement in both major outcomes and rehabilitation. The majority of evidence favours an ability of epidural analgesia to reduce postoperative cardiovascular and pulmonary complications, and there is also consistent evidence that epidural analgesia with LA is associated with faster resolution of postoperative ileus after major abdominal surgery, compared to systemic opioids (Hanna 2009). But while there is evidence favouring epidural analgesia following major surgery in high-risk patients, controversy exists as to whether epidural analgesia also reduces the intensive care resources following major surgery. In a study where patients were followed after thoraco-abdominal oesophagectomy, higher calculated costs of epidural versus systemic pain treatment were outweighed by lower postoperative costs of intensive care, and the overall costs of postoperative care were in fact the same in the two groups (Bartha 2008). In a prospective but non-randomized study on pancreato-duodenectomy, patients receiving epidurals had, surprisingly, significantly higher rates of major complications (pancreatic fistulae, postoperative ileus) and more often required discharge to rehabilitation facilities. Also, 31% of epidural infusions were aborted before anticipated because of haemodynamic compromise or inadequate analgesia (Pratt 2008). Similar adverse events were observed in a study on liver resections; 20% epidurals failed, and patients with epidurals required more intravenous colloid than patients on systemic opioids (Revie 2011). Few individual clinical trials have had sufficient subject numbers to definitively determine the effects of postoperative analgesia on major outcomes. In two comprehensive systematic reviews, the majority of evidence favours an ability of epidural analgesia to reduce postoperative cardiovascular and pulmonary complications only after major vascular surgery or in high-risk patients. However, this finding may become irrelevant because of rapid conversion of major surgery to minimally invasive techniques that carry less risk of complications. There is also consistent evidence that epidural analgesia with local anaesthetics is associated with faster resolution of postoperative ileus after major abdominal surgery, but this finding may also become irrelevant with increasing use of laparoscopic and multimodal fast-track protocols (Liu 2007). No differences were found in mortality, length of stay in hospital, or other morbidity variables (Seller 2008). In yet another exhaustive meta-analysis comparing epidural versus systemic analgesia, the authors found that epidurals carried a reduced risk of pneumonia, independent of site of surgery, catheter insertion, duration of analgesia, or regimen. Epidural analgesia reduced the need for prolonged ventilation or re-intubation, improved lung function and blood oxygenation, but also increased the risk of hypotension, urinary retention, and pruritus. In addition, the beneficial effect on pulmonary function has in fact lessened considerably over the last 35 years because of an overall decrease in the baseline risk (Pöpping 2008). As for the risk of bladder paresis, urinary retention requiring catheterization carries the risk of infection and is generally a problem after abdominal surgery. In a recent meta-analysis, the authors found that the duration of detrusor dysfunction following neuraxial anaesthesia was correlated with LA dose and potency, and the incidence of urinary retention was increased by the presence of neuraxial opioids (Choi 2012).

3.5. Analgesic efficacy of truncal blocks compared to epidural analgesia

There can be no doubt that the administration of continuous epidural analgesia following abdominal surgery has remained - to this day - the golden standard for the provision of post- and perioperative pain management following major abdominal surgery. Only few studies have compared the efficacy of TAP blocks to epidural analgesia. In a matched-control study comparing continuous TAP block catheters to thoracic epidurals, no differences in pain scores were seen over a 3-day follow-up period. Therapeutic failure rate was higher in the epidural group, and the incidence of hypotension was also greater (Kadam 2011). Niraj et al. are also amongst the few having compared the new techniques versus the older and more established techniques (Niraj 2011). Dr. Niraj compared the analgesic efficacy of the subcostal TAP block catheter technique (very much resembling the technique described by Dr. Hebbard) with the epidural analgesia for patients undergoing elective open hepatobiliary or renal surgery. The primary outcome measure was visual analogue pain scores during coughing at 8, 24, 48 and 72 hours after surgery, and they found no significant differences in median VAS during coughing. Tramadol consumption was, however, significantly greater in the TAP group. Very recently, one of the major pioneers of modern regional anaesthesiological practices has published a rather controversial special article (Rawal 2012). The conclusion of the paper is very direct: "It is therefore no exaggeration to suggest that the diminishing role of epidural analgesia can be expected to diminish further. Epidural analgesia remains the gold standard for pain relief in labour because there are currently no good alternatives.This can no longer be said of the use of the epidural analgesia after surgery, and it can therefore no longer be described as the gold standard in postoperative analgesia. The continued use of epidural techniques in your institution should be based on a careful evaluation of its risks and benefits drawn from local audit data, rather than on a tradition that is increasingly being viewed as outdated".

Continuing along this venue of argumentation, a recent study on continuous wound installation after laparotomy found that this method was in fact the most cost-effective compared to epidural or systemic therapy (Tilleul 2012). A pre-peritoneal catheter reduced the demand for epidural analgesia after colonic surgery (Ozturk 2011). Continuous paravertebral nerve blocks provided excellent analgesia after major abdominal or retroperitoneal procedures (Burns 2008). Finally, continuous paravertebral nerve blocks provided better pain at rest and during coughing, less opioid consumption, superior pulmonary function, and were associated with less nausea and hypotension than epidural analgesia in patients undergoing thoracotomy (Davis 2006). Similar benefits of the paravertebral nerve blocks were observed in abdominal, pelvic and urological surgery (Bigler 1989, Burns 2008; Ben-Ari 2009). Although still tentative, these studies suggest that a diverse group of truncal blocks may at the very least be as effective as the epidural block. Some of the physiological effects and potential analgesic and side effects of these techniques are outlined in Table 4. Future research will no doubt be able to enhance our knowledge concerning direct comparison between the various techniques.

Parameter	Epidural block	Truncal block
Physiology		
Lung volumes	Reduced	No change
Postoperative pulmonary dysfunction	Reduced	?
Postoperative pneumonia	Probably reduced	?
Heart frequency	Increased	No change
Blood pressure	Reduced	No change
Coronary blood flow	Increased	?
Myocardial infarction risk	Slightly reduced	?
Splanchnic venous pooling	Increased	Probably no change
Gastrointestinal circulation	Probably increased	?
Postoperative bowel function	Increased if LA alone	?
Urinary bladder paralysis	Yes	No
Perioperative immune suppression	Probably reduced	?
Postoperative rehabilitation		
Postoperative pain	Reduced	Reduced
Continuous analgesia	Yes	Yes, if intermittent boluses or catheter
Prevention of chronic pain	No	?
Opioid demands	Reduced	Reduced
Out-of-bed mobilization	Increased	Probably increased
Side effects and logistics		
Block failure rate	20-30%	10-20%
Lower extremity motor weakness	5-15%	0%
Risk of systemic LA toxicity	Yes	Yes
Risk of neurological damage	Yes	Probably not
Usable during anticoagulation	No	Yes
Pruritus	Yes, if opioids	No

References to Table 4: Liu 1995, Jørgensen 2000, Groeben 2006, Liu 2007, McDonnell 2007, Burns 2008, Clemente 2008, Nakayoshi 2008, Pratt 2008, Jensen 2009, Königsrainer 2009, Børglum 2011, Kadam 2011, Niraj 2011, Petersen 2011.

Table 4. Comparison of the epidural and truncal blocks

Author details

Jens Børglum* and Kenneth Jensen
Copenhagen University Hospital: Bispebjerg,
Department of Anaesthesia and Intensive Care Medicine, Bispebjerg, Denmark

4. References

Abdallah FW, Chan VW, Brull R. Transversus abdominis plane block. A systematic review. Reg Anesth Pain Med 2012; 37: 193-209.

Abrahams MS, Horn J-L, Noles M, Aziz MF. Evidenc-based medicine. Ultrasound guidance for truncal blocks. Reg Anesth Pain Med 2010; 35; S36-S42

Ahlers O, Nachtigall I, Lenze J, Goldmann A, Schulte E, Höhne C, Fritz G, Keh D. Intraoperative thoracic epidural anaesthesia attenuates stress-induced immunosuppression in patients undergoing major abdominal surgery. Br J Anaesth 2008; 101: 781-787

Bacon, DR. Gaston Labat, John Lundy, Emery Rovenstine, and the Mayo Clinic: the spread of regional anesthesia in America between the world wars. Journal of Clinical Anesthesia 2002; 14: 315-320.

Bartha E, Rudin A, Flisberg P, Lundberg CJ, Carlsson P, Kalman S. Could benefits of epidural analgesia following oesophagectomy be measured by perceived perioperative patient workload? Acta Anaesth Scand 2008; 52: 1313-1318

Ben-Ari AY, Moreno GM, Chelly JE, Bigeleisen PE. Ultrasound guided approach for a continuous intercostal approach to the paravertebral space. Anesth Analg 2009; 109: 1691-1694

Berta E, Spanhel J, Smakal O, Smolka V, Gabrhelik T, Lönnqvist PA. Single injection paravertebral block for renal surgery in children. Paediatr Anaesth 2008; 18: 593-597

Bier A. Versuche über cocainisierung des rückenmarkes. Deutsch Zeitschr Chir 1899; 51: 361-368

Bigler D, Dirkes W, Hansen R, Rosenberg J, Kehlet H. Effects of thoracic paravertebral block with bupivacaine vs. combined thoracic epidural block with bupivacaine and morphine on pain and pulmonary function after cholecystectomy. Acta Anaesthesiol Scand 1989; 33: 561-564

Blackford D, Hewitt P, Pande G, Nguyen H, Chilvers C, Robertson I. Future of analgesia for abdominal laparotomy. ANZ J Surg 2008; 78: 527-529

Bunting P, McGeachie JF. Intercostal nerve blockade producing analgesia after appendectomy. Br J Anaesth 1988; 61: 169-172

Burns DA, Ben-David B, Chelly JE, Greensmith JE. Intercostally placed paravertebral catheterization: an alternative approach to continuous paravertebral blockade. Anesth Analg 2008; 107: 339-341

* Corresponding Author

Bærentzen F, Maschmann C, Jensen K, Belhage B, Hensler M, Børglum J. Ultrasound-guided nerve block for inguinal hernia repair: A randomized, controlled double-blinded study. Reg Anesth Pain Med 2012 (Accepted for publication April 2012).

Børglum J, Maschmann C, Belhage B, Jensen K. Ultrasound-guided bilateral dual transversus abdominis plane block: a new four-point approach. Acta Anaesthesiol Scand 2011; 55: 658-663

Børglum J, Jensen K, Christensen AF, Hoegberg LCG, Johansen SS, Lönnqvist P-A, Jansen T. Distribution patterns, dermatomal anesthesia, and ropivacaine serum concentrations after bilateral dual transversus abdominis plane block. Reg Anesth Pain Med 2012; 37: 294-301

Carney J, McDonnell JG, Ochana A, Bhinder R, Laffey JG. The transversus abdominis place block provides effective postoperative analgesia in patients undergoing total abdominal hysterectomy. Anesth Analg 2008; 107: 2056-2060

Carney J, Finnerty O, Rauf J, Curley G, McDonnell JG, Laffey JG. Ipsilateral transversus abdominis plane block provides effective analgesia after appendectomy in children: a randomized controlled trial. Anesth Analg 2010; 111: 998-1003

Carney J, Finnerty O, Rauf J, Bergin D, Laffey JG, McDonnel JG. Studies on the spread of local anaesthetic solution in transversus abdominis plane blocks. Anaesthesia 2011; 66: 1023-1030.

Catro-Alves LJ, De Azevedo VL, De Freitas Braga TF, Goncalves AC, De Oliveira GS. The effect of neuraxial versus general anesthesia techniques on postoperative quality of recovery and analgesia after abdominal hysterectomy: a prospective, randomized, controlled trial. Anesth Analg 2011; 113: 1480-1486

Choi S, Mahon P, Awad IT. Neuraxial anesthesia and bladder dysfunction in the perioperative period: a systematic review. Can J Anaesth 2012 [Epub ahead of print]

Clemente A, Carli F. The physiological effects of thoracic epidural anesthesia and analgesia on the cardiovascular, respiratory and gastrointestinal systems. Minerva Anestesiol 2008; 74: 549-563

Côté AV, Vachon CA, Horlocker TT, Bacon DR.From Victor Pauchet to Gaston Labat: The Transformation of Regional Anesthesia from a Surgeon's Practice to the Physician Anesthesiologist. Anesth Analg 2003; 96: 1193-1200

Davies RG, Myles PS, Graham JM. A comparison of the analgesic efficacy and side-effects of paravertebral vs. epidural blockade for thoracotomy: a systematic review and meta-analysis of randomized trials. Br J Anesth 2006; 96: 418-426

Dolan J, Lucie P, Geary T, Smith M, Kenny GN. The rectus sheath block: accuracy of local anesthetic placement by trainee anesthesiologists using loss of resistance or ultrasound guidance. Reg Anesth Pain Med 2009; 34: 247-250

El-Dawlatly AA, Trkistani A, Kettner SC, Machata A.-M., Delvi MB, Thallaj A, Kapral S, Marhofer P. Ultrasound-guided transversus abdominis plane block: description of a new technique and comparison with conventional systemic analgesia during laparoscopic cholecystectomy. Br J Anaesth 2009; 109: 763-767

Eichenberger U, Greher M, Kirchmair L, Curatolo M, Moriggl B. Ultrasound-guided blocks of the ilioinguinal and iliohypogastric nerve: accuracy of a selective new technique confirmed by anatomical dissection. Br J Anaesth 2006;97:238-243

Ferguson S, Thomas V, Lewis I. The rectus sheath block in paediatric anaesthesia: new indications for an old technique? Paediatr Anaesth 1996; 6: 463-466

Fujita Y, Horiguchi Y, Nakamura K, Ikeda D, Kaneko M, Tomioka K, Tokunaga C, Iwakura T. Effect of postoperative analgesia by repeated transversus abdominis plane blocks via a placed catheter in patients undergoing ovarian cystectomy. Masui 2012; 61: 155-158

Groeben H. Epidural anesthesia and pulmonary function. J Anesth 2006; 20: 290-299

Hanna MN, Murphy JD, Kumar K, Wu CL. Regional techniques and outcome: what is the evidence? Curr Opin Anaesthesiol 2009; 22: 672-677

Hebbard PD, Barrington MJ, Vasey C. Ultrasound-guided continuous oblique subcostal transversus abdominis plane blockade: description of anatomy and clinical technique. Reg Anesth Pain Med 2010; 35: 436-441

Hivelin M, Wyniecki A, Plaud B, Marty J, Lantieri L. Ultrasound-guided bilateral transversus abdominis plane block for postoperative analgesia after breast reconstruction DIEP flap. Plast Reconstr Surg 2011; 128: 44-55

Ho AM, Karmakar MK, Cheung M, Lam GC. Right thoracic paravertebral analgesia for hepatectomy. Br J Anaesth 2004; 93:458-461

Jensen K, Børglum J. Predictors of failure of interscalene nerve blocks for shoulder surgery. A 4-year cohort study. Reg Anesth Pain Med 2011; 36: 508-520

Jensen K, Børglum J. The fate of the epidurals. European Society of Regional Anaesthesia, 31st Congress, Bordeaux 2012 (Submitted)

Jensen K, Børglum J. Ultrasound-guided quadratus lumborum block with a curved probe for a morbidly obese patient. European Society of Regional Anaesthesia, 2012 Congress, Bordeaux (Submitted)

Jensen K, Kehlet H, Lund CM. Postoperative recovery profile after elective abdominal hysterectomy: a prospective, observational study of a multimodal anaesthetic regime. Eur J Anaesth 2009; 26: 382-388

Jørgensen H, Wetterslev J, Møiniche S, Dahl JB. Epidural local anaesthetics versus opioid-based analgesic regimens on postoperative gastrointestinal paralysis, PONV and pain after abdominal surgery. Cochrane Database Syst Rev 2000: CD 001893

Kadam VR, Moran JL. Epidural infusions versus transversus abdominis plane (TAP) block infusions: retrospective study. J Anesth 2011; 25: 786-787

Kamarkar MK. Thoracic paravertebral block. Anesthesiology 2001; 95: 771-780

Knowles P, Hancox D, Letheren M, Eddleston J. An evaluation of intercostal nerve blockade for analgesia following renal transplantation. Eur J Anaesthesiol 1998; 15: 457-461

Koscielniak-Nielsen ZJ. Transversus abdominis plane blocks for rescue analgesia after major abdominal surgery. Acta Anaesthesiol Scand 2011; 55: 635-637

Kortgen AM, Silomon M, Pape-Becker C, Buchinger H, Grundmann U, Bauer M.l Thoracic but not lumbar epidural anaesthesia increases liver blood flow after major abdominal surgery. Eur J Anaesth 2009; 26: 111-116

Königsrainer I, Bredanger S, Drewel-Frohnmeyer R, Vonthein R, Krueger WA, Königsrainer A, Unerti KE, Schroeder TH. Audit of motor weakness and premature catheter dislodgement after epidural analgesia in major abdominal surgery. Anaesthesia 2009; 64: 27-31

Labat G. Regional anaesthesia. Its technique and clinical application. WB Saunders, New York 1922

Liu SS, Carpenter RL, Neal JM. Epidural anesthesia and analgesia their role in postoperative outcome. Anesthesiology 1995; 82: 1474-1506

Liu SS, Wu CL. Effect of postoperative analgesia on major postoperative complications: a systematic update of the evidence. Anesth Analg 2007; 104: 689-702

Lund C, Hansen OB, Kehlet H, Mogensen T, Qvitzau S. Effects of etidocaine administered epidurally on changes in somatosensory evoked potentials after dermatomal stimulation. Reg Anesth 1991; 16: 38-42

McDonnell J, O'Donnell B, Tuite D, Farrell T, Power C. The regional abdominal field infiltration (R.A.F.I.) technique: computerized tomographic and anatomical identification of a novel approach to the transversus abdominis neuro-vascular fascial plane. Anesthesiology 2004; 101: A899

McDonnell J, O'Donnell B, Farrell T, Gough N, Tuite D, Power C, Laffey J. Transversus abdominis plane block: a cadaveric and radiological evaluation. Reg Anesth Pain Med 2007; 32: 399-404

Moussa AA. Opioid saving strategy: bilateral single-site thoracic paravertebral block in right lobe donor hepatectomy. Middle East J Anesthesiol 2008; 19: 789-801

Nakayoshi T, Kawasaki N, Suzuki Y, Urashima M, Hanyu N, Yanaga K. Epidural analgesia and gastrointestinal motility after open abdominal surgery – a review. J Smooth Muscle Res 2008; 44: 57-64

Naja MZ, Ziade MF, Lönnqvist PA. Bilateral paravertebral somatic nerve block for ventral hernia repair. Eur J Anaesthesiol 2002, 19: 197-202.

Naja MZ, Ziade MF, El Rajab M, El Tayara K, Lönnqvist PA. Varying anatomical injection points within the thoracic paravertebral space: effect on spread of solution and nerve blockade. Anaesthesia 2004; 59: 459–463

Narinder R. Epidural Technique for Postoperative Pain. Gold Standard No More? Reg Anesth Pain Med 2012; 37: 310-317

Niraj G, Kelkar A, Jeyapalan I, Graff-Baker P, w-illiamas O, Darbar A, Maheshwaran A, Powell R. Comparison of analgesic efficacy of subcostal transversus abdominus plane blocks with epidural analgesia following upper abdominal surgeryAnaesthesia 2011; 66: 465-471

Niraj G, Kelkar A, Fox AJ. Oblique sub-costal transversus abdominis plane (TAP) catheters: an alternative to epidural analgesia after upper abdominal surgery. Anaesthesia 2009; 64: 1137-1140

Orebaugh SL et al. Interscalene block using ultrasound guidance: impact of experience on resident performance. Acta Anaesth Scand 2009; 53: 1268-1274

Osaka Y, Kashiwagi M, Nagatsuka Y, Oosaku M, Hirose C. Ultrasound-guided rectus sheath block for upper abdominal surgery. Masui 2010; 59: 1039-1041

Ozturk E, Yilmazlar A, Coskun F, Isik O, Yilmazlar T. The beneficial effects of preperitoneal catheter analgesia following colon and rectal resections: a prospective, randomized, double-blind, placebo-controlled study. Tech Coloproctol 2011; 15: 331-336

Panaretou V, Toufektzian L, Siafaka I, Kouroukli I, Sigala F, Vlachopoulos C, Katsaragakis S, Zografos G, Filis K. Postoperative pulmonary function after open abdominal aortic aneurysm repair in patients with chronic obstructive pulmonary disease: epidural versus intravenous analgesia. Ann Vasc Surg 2012; 26: 149-155.

Papadima A, Boutsikou M, Lagoudianakis EE, Kataki A, Konstadoulakis M, Georgiou L, Katergiannakis V, Manouras A. Lymphocyte apoptosis after major abdominal surgery is not influenced by anesthetic technique: a comparative study of general anesthesia versus combined general and epidural analgesia. J Clin Anesth 2009; 21: 414-421

Petersen PL, Mathiesen O, Thorup H, Dahl JB. The transversus abdominis plane block: a valuable option for post-operative analgesia? A topical review. Acta Anaesthesiol Scand 2010; 54: 529-539

Petersen M, Elers J, Børglum J, Belhage B, Mortensen J, Maschmann C. Is Pulmonary Function Affected by Bilateral Dual Transversus Abdominis Plane Block? A Randomized,Placebo-Controlled, Double-Blind, Crossover Pilot Study in Healthy Male Volunteers. Reg Anesth Pain Med 2011; 36: 568-571

Pratt WB, Steinbrook RA, Maithel SK, Vanounou T, Callery MP, Vollmer CM. Epidural analgesia for pancreatoduodenectomy: a critical appraisal. J Gastrointest Surg 2008; 12: 1207-1220

Pöpping DM, Elia N, Marret E, Remy C, Tramer MR. Protective effects of epidural analgesia on pulmonary complications after abdominal and thoracic surgery: a meta-analysis. Arch Surg 2008; 143: 990-999

Rafi AN. Abdominal field block: a new approach via the lumbar triangle. Anaesthesia. 2001; 56: 1024-1026

Renes SH, Bruhn J, Gielen MJ, Scheffer GJ, Van Geffen GJ. In-Plane Ultrasound-Guided Thoracic Paravertebral Block. A Preliminary Report of 36 Cases With Radiologic Confirmation of Catheter Position. Reg Anesth Pain Med 2010; 35: 212-216

Revie EJ, Massie LJ, McNally SJ, McKeown DW, Garden OJ, Wigmore SJ. Effectiveness of epidural analgesia following open liver resection. HPB (Oxford); 13: 206-211

Rodgers A, Walker N, Schug S, McKee A, Kehlet H, van Zundert A, Sage D, Futter M, Saville G, Clark T, MacMahon S. Reduction of postoperative mortality and morbidity with epidural or spinal anaesthesia: results from overview of randomised trials. BMJ 2000; 321: 1493-1505

Rozen WM, Tran TMN, Ashton MW, Barrington MJ, Ivanusic JJ, Taylor GI. Refining the Course of the thoracolumbar nerves: A new understanding of the innervation of the anterior abdominal wall. Clin Anat 2008, 21: 325-333

Seller Losada JM, Sifre Julio C, Ruiz Garcia V. Rev Esp Anestesiol Reanim 2008; 55: 360-366

Shin HJ, Kim ST, Yim KH, Lee HS, Sim JH, Shin YD. Preemptive analgesic efficacy of ultrasound-guided transversus abdominis plane block in patients undergoing gynecologic surgery via a transverse lower abdominal skin incision. Korean J Anesth 2011; 61: 413-418

Shibata Y, Sato Y, Fujiwara Y, Komatsu T. Transversus abdominis plane block. Anesth Analg 2007; 105:883

Siddiqui MR, Sajid MS, Uncles DR, Cheek L, Baig MK. A meta-analysis on the clinical effectiveness of transversus abdominis plane block. J Clin Anesth 2011; 23: 7-14

Siriussawakul A, Mandee S, Thonsontia J, Vitayaburananont P, Areewatana S, Laonarinthawoot J. Obesity, epidural analgesia, and subcostal incision are risk factors for postoperative desaturation. Can J Anaesth 2010; 57: 415-422

Sites BD, Chan VW, Neal JM, Weller R, Grau T, Koscielniak-Nielsen ZJ, Ivani G. The American Society of Regional Anesthesia and Pain Medicine and the European Society of Regional Anaesthesia and Pain Therapy joint committee recommendations for education and training in ultrasound-guided regional anesthesia. Reg Anesth Pain Med. 2010, 35(2): 74-80

Thompson JE. An anatomical and experimental study of sacral anaesthesia Ann Surg 1917; 66: 718-727

Tilleul P, Aissou M, Bocquet F, Thiriat N, le Grelle O, Burke MJ, Hutton J, Beaussier M. Cost-effectiveness analysis comparing epidural, patient-controlled intravenous morphine, and continuous wound infiltration for postoperative pain management after open abdominal surgery. Br J Anaesth 2012 (Epub ahead of print)

Van Lier F, van der Geest PJ, Hoeks SE, van Gestel YR, Hol JW, Sin DD, Stolker RJ, Poldermans D. Epidural analgesia is associated with improved health outcomes of surgical patients with chronic obstructive pulmonary disease. Anesthesiology 2011; 115: 315-321

Vieira AM, Schnaider TP, Brandao AC, Campos Neto JP. Comparative study of intercostal and interpleural block for post-cholecystectomy analgesia. Rev Bras Anestesiol 2003; 53: 346-350

Weintraud M, Marhofer P, Bosenberg A et al. Ilioinguinal/iliohypogastric blocks in children: where do we administer the local anesthetic without direct visualization? Anesth Analg 2008; 106:89-93

Willschke H, Bosenberg A, Marhofer P, Johnston S, Kettner S, Eichenberger U, Wanzel O, Kapral S. Ultrasonographic-guided ilioinguinal/iliohypogastric nerve block in pediatric anesthesia: what is the optimal volume? Anesth Analg 2006;102: 1680-1684

Willschke H, Marhofer P, Bosenberg A, Johnston S, Wanzel O, Cox S G, Sitzwohl C, Kapral S. Ultrasonography for ilioinguinal/Iliohypo-gastric nerve blocks in children. Br J Anaesth 2005;95:226-230

Wolf AR. Effects of regional analgesia on stress responses to pediatric surgery. Paediatr Anaesth 2012; 22: 19-24

Young MJ, Gorlin AW, Modest VE, Quarishi SA. Clinical implications of the transversus abdominis plane block in adults. Anesthesiol Res Pract 2012 (Epub ahead of print)

Chapter 4

Study of Vitamin C Administration Effect on Postoperative Plasma IL-6 Concentrations in Septic Patients After Abdominal Surgery

Ignacio Ferrón-Celma, Carmen Olmedo, Alfonso Mansilla,
Ana Garcia-Navarro, Karim Muffak, Pablo Bueno and Jose-Antonio Ferrón

Additional information is available at the end of the chapter

http://dx.doi.org/10.5772/48676

1. Introduction

Satisfactory post-surgical recovery is reflected in a reduction in plasma levels of pro-inflammatory and anti-inflammatory cytokines, which are higher in septic and surgery patients than in healthy individuals [1-4]. The persistence of inflammatory cytokines in the circulation indicates a generalized systemic inflammatory response and is associated with Multiple-Organ Dysfunction Syndrome (MODS) and death in critically ill patients [5].

In the systemic inflammatory response, inflammation and coagulation can be stimulated by microbial invasion (exogenous injury) or direct tissue injury (endogenous injury), when the NF-kB protein translocates into the nucleus and activates the transcription of both proinflammatory (e.g. IL-6) and anti-inflammatory (e.g. IL-10) cytokines [6].

In the course of an inflammatory process, endothelial cells and polymorphonuclear leukocytes (PMNs) generate elevated amounts of reactive oxygen species (ROS) [7], which act as secondary mediators, inducing chemotactic substances (e.g. cytokines) and adhesion molecules that amplify the inflammatory process. Vitamin C is a hydrosoluble antioxidant molecule that acts as ROS scavenger and vitamin E regenerator [8] and has been shown to reduce cytokine production in different assays [9-12].

The microcirculation is particularly susceptible to oxidative stress which leads to the systemic inflammatory response syndrome, hemodynamic instability, and multiple organ failure [13]. Vitamin C plasma concentrations are strongly altered in patients with sepsis [14]. Restoring antioxidant and endothelial functions in the critically ill patient requires supraphysiologic concentrations of ascorbate [15]. Such concentrations can only be achieved by parenteral administration. In a trial in 14 patients, 2 days on 3000 mg/d given intravenously were required in critically ill patients to obtain a significant increase of plasma ascorbate concentrations [16]. The rapid replenishment of ascorbate is of special clinical significance in critically ill patients because these patients experience drastic reductions in ascorbate concentrations, and this may be a causal factor in the development of circulatory shock [17]. In a randomized controlled antioxidant trial including 200 patients in the ICU and providing a combination of selenium, zinc, vitamin C, and vitamin B1, it was shown no survival benefit, but antioxidants shortened hospital stay in surviving trauma patients [18]. In a retrospective trial involving 4294 patients, of whom 2272 received antioxidants for 7 days, resulted in a 28% relative risk reduction in mortality and a significant reduction in both hospital and ICU length of stay [19].

The rationale for a benefit in this category of patients with requirements for major wound healing is strong and is reinforced by the beneficial effects shown in the trials that included vitamin C. The optimal duration of supplementation has not yet been determined, but benefits appear after 5 days of supplementation. On the basis of the pharmacokinetic aspects of antioxidants, an intravenous dose ranging between 1 and 3 g/d should probably be considered independent of parenteral nutrition doses in patients with major trauma at least during the first week after injury [17].

Cytokines exert a key role in inflammatory host defense, therefore the study of their levels and their pharmacological modulation is of great interest for the management of septic patients who underwent abdominal surgery.

2. Patients and methods

2.1. Study design and patients: A prospective, pilot study was performed in 20 consecutive septic abdominal surgery patients in our Digestive Surgery Department with postoperative mortality risk of >30 % by POSSUM score [20]. POSSUM was selected to predict death rate more accurately compared to the APACHE II classification [21]. In all cases, sepsis was produced by peritoneal infection. Patient characteristics are listed in Table 1. Ten healthy volunteers were recruited as a control group. Written informed consent was obtained from all patients or their relatives, and the study was approved by the local Clinical Research Ethics Committee. Allocation of patients to experimental (n=10) or placebo (n=10) group was by envelope randomization (designed by a statistician).

2.2. Treatments: Experimental and placebo treatments were started at 12 h post-surgery. Treatments were administered daily on 6 consecutive postoperative days. The experimental (vitamin C) group received 450 mg/day of the vitamin in 5% dextrose administered in three equal doses, and the placebo group received an identical administration of 5% dextrose following previous studies [22,23]. Placebo-treated patients received no supplemental nutrition containing vitamins nor vitamin C.

2.2. Samples: Early-morning peripheral blood samples were drawn for 7-9 a.m. by venipuncture from all patients on every treatment day into a 3-ml sterile EDTA tube. They were immediately centrifuged at room temperature (400 x g for 16 min), and the supernatant (plasma) was taken for cytokine determination. Sample collection started at 24 h after vitamin C/placebo administration (T1d) and lasted for 6 days (T1d, T2d, T3d, T4d, T5d and T6d).

2.4. Measurements: Plasma IL-6 concentrations were determined in a FACScan flow cytometer (Becton Dickinson, San Jose, CA, USA) using the BD Cytometric Bead Array (CBA) (Becton Dickinson, San Jose, CA, USA). The CBA technique employs a series of particles with discrete fluorescence intensities to simultaneously detect soluble analytes [24]. The BD CBA system uses the sensitivity of amplified fluorescence detection by flow cytometry to measure soluble analytes in a particle-based immunoassay. Each bead in a BD CBA provides a capture surface for a specific protein and is analogous to an individually coated well in an ELISA plate. The sensitivity of the BD CBA system was 3.0 pg/ml for IL-6.

2.5. Statistical analysis: A two-way analysis of variance was performed between quantitative independent variables (plasma cytokine concentrations) and qualitative dependent variables (placebo/Vitamin C treatment). Because of the small number of patients in each treatment group, a non-parametric test (U Mann-Whitney) was applied to compare differences between the treatment groups and between these groups and the healthy controls. $P<0.05$ was considered significant. Data are presented as mean values ± standard error (SE).

3. Results

General characteristics of patients are listed in Table 1. Four (40%) of the ten patients in each group (vitamin C and placebo) developed MODS during the 6 days postoperative period studied. At the end of this period, the postoperative mortality rate was 40% in the placebo group and 60% in the vitamin C group.

Plasma IL-6 concentrations were significantly reduced in experimental group, which received vitamin C, compared with the placebo group during most of the postoperative period, reaching a significant difference on day 2 and day 6 (p=0.048 and p=0.033) (Figure 1). Table 2 shows IL-6 values during 6the period of study.

	PLACEBO (n=10)	**Vitamin C (n=10)**
Age (years)	65.1 ± 3.6	67.8 ± 4.5
Mortality risk: %	52.0 ± 4.1	60.5 ± 8.7
POSSUM: Score	50.4 ± 1.4	55.0 ± 3.3
Sex (Men/Women)	6/4	5/5
Diagnoses		
Peritonitis (perforations or inflammations of gallbladder, colon, biliary or cholecystitis and ulcers)	6	7
Complicated intestinal ischemia	1	1
Intra-abdominal abscesses	1	1
Anastomotic leakage after gastrectomy	1	0
Cholangitis	1	1

Surgical Procedure		
Intestinal resection with or without anastomosis	5	3
Perforation suture	3	3
Collection drainage or anastomosis dehiscence	1	1
Cholecystectomy with or without drainage of biliary tract	1	3
Pressors	2/10	3/10
Ventilatory support	2/10	3/10
Oxygenation Parameters PO_2 (mmHg)	144.7± 47.3	113.9 ±50.5
Oxygenation Parameters PCO_2 (mmHg)	47.2 ± 7.4	45.7 ± 7.7
Creatinine (mg/dl)	1.99 ± 0.21	2.15 ± 0.12
Lactate (meq/L)	1.97 ± 0.55	3.22 ±1.25
Volume Status (based on the blood sodium level in mmol/L)	137.42 ±7.19	138.07±6.11

Table 1. General characteristics, diagnoses and surgical procedures of abdominal surgery patients studied. Data are presented as mean values ± standard error of mean (SEM).

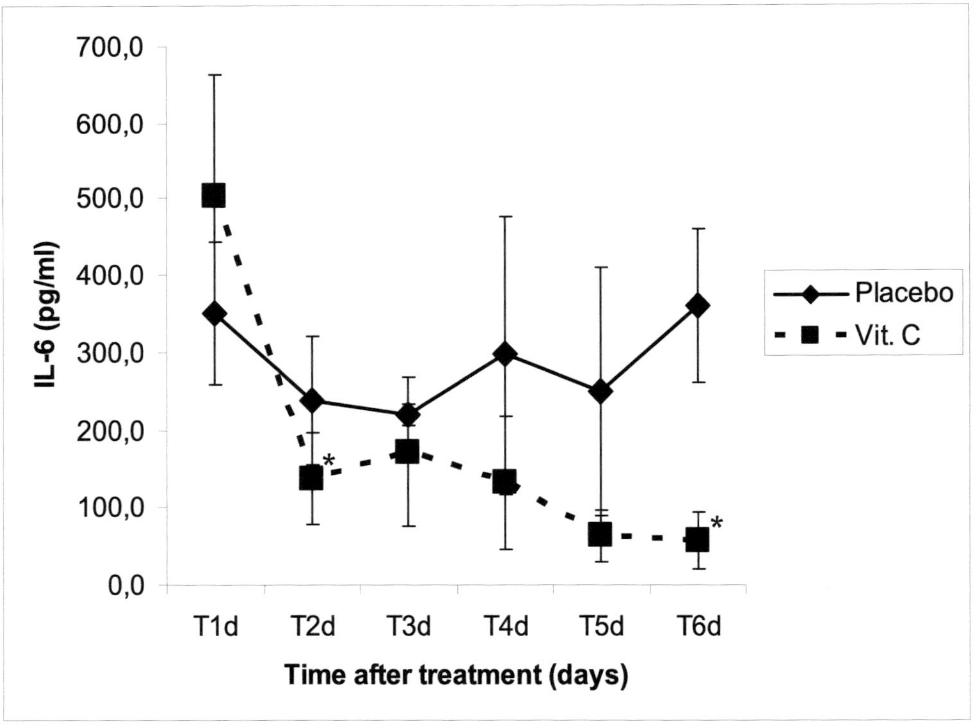

Figure 1. Time course of plasma IL-6 levels (pg/ml) in vitamin C and placebo-treated surgical patients. Statistically significant differences are marked with asterisk (T2d: p=0.048, T6d: p=0.033).

Cytokine	Healthy Control	Group	T1d	T2d	T3d	T4d	T5d	T6d
IL-6 (pg/ml)	9.7 ± 2.4	Placebo	350.5 ± 92.6	237.5 ± 82.3	219.3 ± 13.2	296.3 ± 78.5	248.9 ±159.6	359.7 ± 99.9
		Vit. C	502.3 ±161.3	136.4 ± 59.3	171.4 ± 95.5	132.5 ± 85.8	63.0 ± 34.2	57.1 ± 36.2

Table 2. IL-6 values (pg/ml) in placebo and vitamin C groups.

4. Discussion

Plasma IL-6 high concentrations have been documented in high-risk septic abdominal surgery patients [1, 25, 26]. Elevated plasma cytokine levels derive from severe inflammatory processes caused by the disease resulting in an excess of inflammatory mediators. Taking into account the severity of the inflammatory process, plasma cytokine levels have been related to post-surgical complications [4, 25, 26, 27], organ dysfunction development [5, 25, 28, 29] and mortality in critical care, surgery, sepsis and SIRS [1, 3, 29, 30-35]. These events are related to the pro-inflammatory environment that predominates in sepsis, which is responsible for the overactivation of leukocytes and endothelial cells associated with tissue injury. Elevated levels of pro-inflammatory cytokines, notably IL-6, produce early PMN priming and sequestration and are potential mediators of early tissue damage [36,37], exacerbating systemic inflammation through the chronic release of toxic products at inflammation sites [38]. The results presented in our study in patients who underwent abdominal surgery, demonstrate that vitamin C has an inhibitory effect on plasma cytokine concentrations, finding lower IL-6 levels in the vitamin-treated versus placebo-treated patients that reached significance after 2 days and 6 days of treatment. These observations are according with those previously reported for *in vitro* studies by Härtel et al [9] and Bergman et al [10], in studies describing the effect of vitamin C on the intracytoplasmic production of pro-inflammatory cytokines in whole blood samples of healthy individuals, and *in vivo* by Fischer et al [11] reporting that supplementation with antioxidants in healthy volunteers inhibited the IL-6 release from the contracting human skeletal muscle.

The results showed in the present report contribute to clarify the optimal duration of supplementation and reinforce the concept that benefits appear after 5 days of supplementation such as has been noted previously [17].

This inhibitory effect of vitamin C on cytokine production may result from a reduction in the production of ROS, which are at least in part responsible for excessive cytokine production by promoting cell overproduction or by modulating nuclear factors such as NF-kβ, which is involved in cytokine synthesis [7]. The present findings suggest that ROS clearance by scavengers, such as vitamin C, attenuates plasma levels of IL-6, one of the main pro-inflammatory mediators in the acute inflammatory processes observed in septic patients who underwent abdominal surgery and other critically ill patients. A reduction in plasma IL-6 concentrations may improve the prognosis in patients with postoperative persistence of elevated pro-inflammatory mediators, and has been defined as the best parameter for predicting development of MODS as compared to other cytokines [38].

Although different surgical approaches were used in these patients, according to the decision of the surgeons in charge, we emphasize that all patients had a clinical picture of severe peritonitis and a POSSUM score > 50 points. In our view, the differences in surgical procedure would not have influenced results, although a study of a larger sample of patients is warranted to confirm these results.

In conclusion, further studies in larger patient samples are required to establish whether this pharmacological intervention enhances post-surgery recovery, preventing complications and MODS in septic patients who underwent abdominal surgery.

5. Conclusion

Septic patients who underwent abdominal surgery treated with vitamin C for 6 days post-surgery showed a significant reduction in plasma IL-6 levels, which may benefit these patients by downregulating their enhanced systemic pro-inflammatory response.

Author details

Ignacio Ferrón-Celma, Carmen Olmedo and Pablo Bueno
Experimental Surgery Research Unit, Virgen de las Nieves University Hospital, Granada, Spain

Alfonso Mansilla, Ana Garcia-Navarro, Karim Muffak and Jose-Antonio Ferrón
General and Digestive Surgery Department, Virgen de las Nieves University Hospital, Granada, Spain

Acknowledgement

The authors thank the surgeons and nurses of the General and Digestive Surgery Department and the personnel of the Emergency and Critical Care Department of Virgen de las Nieves University Hospital (Granada, Spain) for their help in patient recruitment and blood sampling. The contribution of pharmacists from the Pharmacy Department of Virgen de las Nieves University Hospital is gratefully acknowledged, as is the excellent technical assistance of the staff of the Experimental Surgery Research Unit and statisticians from the FIBAO foundation.

6. References

[1] Torre D, Tambini R, Aristodemo S, Gavazzeni G, Goglio A, Cantamessa C, Pugliese A, Biondi G. Anti-inflammatory response of IL-4, IL-10 and TGF-beta in patients with systemic inflammatory response syndrome. Mediators Inflamm 2000; 9: 193-5.

[2] Munster AM. Gut: Clinical importance of bacterial translocation, permeability, and other factors. In: Baue AE, Faist E, Fry DE, editors. Multiple Organ Failure: Pathophysiology, prevention and therapy. New York: Springer; 2000. p. 86-1.

[3] Casey LC, Balk RA, Bone RC. Plasma cytokine and endotoxin levels correlate with survival in patients with the sepsis syndrome. Ann Intern Med 1993; 119: 771-8.

[4] Miyaoka K, Iwase M, Suzuki R, Kondo G, Watanabe H, Ito D, et al. Clinical evaluation of circulating interleukin-6 and interleukin-10 levels after surgery-induced inflammation. J Surg Res 2005; 125: 144-50.

[5] Pinsky MR, Vincent JL, Deviere J, Alegre M, Kahn RJ, Dupont E. Serum cytokine levels in human septic shock. Relation to multiple-system organ failure and mortality. Chest 1993; 103: 565-75.

[6] Colmes CL, Russell JA, Walley KB. Geentic polymorphisms in sepsis and septic shock. Chest 2003; 124:1103-15.

[7] Closa D, Folch-Puy E. Oxygen free radicals and the systemic inflammatory response. IUBMB Life. 2004; 56: 185-91.

[8] Goode HF, Webster NR. Free radicals and antioxidants in sepsis. Crit. Care Med. 1993; 21: 1770-6.

[9] Härtel C, Strunk T, Bucsky P, Schultz C. Effects of vitamin C on intracytoplasmic cytokine production in human whole blood monocytes and lymphocytes. Cytokine 2004; 27: 101-6.

[10] Bergman M, Salman H, Djaldetti M, Fish L, Punsky I, Bessler H. In vitro immune response of human peripheral blood cells to vitamins C and E. J Nutr Biochem 2004 15: 45-50.

[11] Fischer CP, Hiscock NJ, Penkowa M, Basu S, Vessby B, Kallner A, et al. Supplementation with vitamins C and E inhibits the release of interleukin-6 from contracting human skeletal muscle. J Physiol 2004; 558: 633-45.

[12] Vassilakopoulos T, Karatza MH, Katsaounou P, Kollintza A, Zakynthinos S, Roussos C. Antioxidants attenuate the plasma cytokine response to exercise in humans. J Appl Physiol 2003; 94: 1025-32.

[13] Biesalski HK, McGregor GP. Antioxidant therapy in critical care–is the microcirculation the primary target? Crit Care Med 2007; 35(Suppl):S577–S583.

[14] Galley HF, Davies MJ, Webster NR. Ascorbyl radical formation in patients with sepsis: effect of ascorbate loading. Free Radic Biol Med 1996;20:139–143.

[15] McGregor GP, Biesalski HK. Rationale and impact of vitamin C in clinical nutrition. Curr Opin Clin Nutr Metab Care 2006;9:697–703.

[16] Long CL, Maull KI, Krishnan RS, et al. Ascorbic acid dynamics in the seriously ill and injured. J Surg Res 2003;109:144–148.

[17] Berger MM. Vitamin C Requirements in Parenteral Nutrition. Gastroenterology 2009; 137: S70-S78.

[18] Berger MM, Soguel L, Shenkin A, et al. Influence of early antioxidant supplements on clinical evolution and organ function in critically ill cardiac surgery, major trauma and subarachnoid hemorrhage patients. Crit Care 2008;12:R101.

[19] Collier BR, Giladi A, Dossett LA, Dyer L, Fleming SB, Cotton BA. Impact of high-dose antioxidants on outcomes in acutely injured patients. J Parenter Enteral Nutr 2008; 32:384–388.

[20] Copeland GP, Jones D, Walters M. POSSUM: a scoring system for surgical audit. Br J Surg 1991; 78: 355-60.

[21] Crea N, Di Fabio F, Pata G, Nascimbeni R. APACHE II, POSSUM, and ASA scores and the risk of perioperative complications in patients with colorectal disease. Ann Ital Chir. 2009; 80(3): 177-81.

[22] Clemens MR, Waladkhani AR, Bublitz K, Ehninger G, Gey KF. Supplementation with antioxidants prior to bone marrow transplantation. Wien Klin Wochenschr 1997; 109: 771-6.

[23] Ferrón-Celma I., Mansilla A., Hassan L., García-Navarro A., Comino A.M., Bueno P., Ferrón J.A. Effect of vitamin C administration on neutrophil apoptosis in septic patients after abdominal surgery. Journal of Surgical Research 2009; 153:2: 224-230.
[24] Cook EB, Stahl JL, Lowe L, Chen R, Morgan E, Wilson J, et al. Simultaneous measurement of six cytokines in a single sample of human tears using microparticle-based flow cytometry: allergics vs. non-allergics. J Immunol Methods 2001; 254: 109-18.
[25] Davis MG, Hagen PO. Systemic inflamatory response syndrome. Br J Surg 1997; 84: 929-35.
[26] Oda S, Hirasawa H, Shiga H, Nakanishi K, Matsuda K, Nakamua M. Sequential measurement of IL-6 blood levels in patients with systemic inflammatory response syndrome (SIRS)/sepsis. Cytokine 2005; 29: 169-175.
[27] Mokart D, Capo C, Blache JL, Delpero JR, Houvenaeghel G, Martin C, et al. Early postoperative compensatory anti-inflammatory response syndrome is associated with septic complications after major surgical trauma in patients with cancer. Br J Surg 2002; 89: 1450-6.
[28] Mokart D, Merlin M, Sannini A, Brun JP, Delpero JR, Houvenaeghel G, et al. Procalcitonin, interleukin 6 and systemic inflammatory response syndrome (SIRS): early markers of postoperative sepsis after major surgery. Br J Anaesth 2005; 94: 767-73.
[29] Friedman G, Jankowski S, Marchant A, Goldman M, Kahn RJ, Vincent JL. Blood interleukin 10 levels parallel the severity of septic shock. J Crit Care 1997; 12: 183-7.
[30] Roumen RM, Hendriks T, van der Ven-Jongekrijg J, Nieuwenhuijzen GA, Sauerwein RW, van der Meer JW, et al. Cytokine patterns in patients after major vascular surgery, hemorrhagic shock, and severe blunt trauma. Relation with subsequent adult respiratory distress syndrome and multiple organ failure. Ann Surg 1993; 218: 769-76.
[31] Van der Poll T, de Waal Malefyt R, Coyle SM, Lowry SF. Antiinflammatory cytokine responses during clinical sepsis and experimental endotoxemia: sequential measurements of plasma soluble interleukin (IL)-1 receptor type II, IL-10, and IL-13. J Infect Dis 1997; 175: 118-22.
[32] Waage A, Halstensen A, Espevik T. Association between tumour necrosis factor in serum and fatal outcome in patients with meningococcal disease. Lancet 1987; 1: 355-7.
[33] Grau GE, Taylor TE, Molyneux ME, Wirima JJ, Vassalli P, Hommel M, et al. Tumor necrosis factor and disease severity in children with falciparum malaria. N Engl J Med 1989; 320: 1586-91.
[34] Debets JM, Kampmeijer R, van der Linden MP, Buurman WA, van der Linden CJ. Plasma tumor necrosis factor and mortality in critically ill septic patients. Crit Care Med 1989; 17: 489-94.
[35] Hack CE, De Groot ER, Felt-Bersma RJ, Nuijens JH, Strack Van Schijndel RJ, Eerenberg-Belmer AJ, et al. Increased plasma levels of interleukin-6 in sepsis. Blood 1989; 74: 1704-10.
[36] Botha AJ, Moore FA, Moore EE, Kim FJ, Banerjee A, Peterson VM, et al. Postinjury neutrophil priming and activation: an early vulnerable window. Surgery 1995; 118: 358-64.
[37] Taniguchi T, Koido Y, Aiboshi J, Yamashita T, Suzaki S, Kurokawa A. Change in the ratio of interleukin-6 to interleukin-10 predicts a poor outcome in patients with systemic inflammatory response syndrome. Crit Care Med 1999; 27: 1262-4.
[38] Frink M, Van Griensven M, Kobbe P, Brin T, Zeckey C, Vaske B, Krettek C, Hildebrand F. IL-6 predicts organ dysfunction and mortality in patients with multiple injuries. Scandinavian Journal of Trauma, Resuscitation and Emergency Medicine 2009; 17:49 doi:10.1186/1757-7241-17-49

Section 3

Contribution of Surgery for Benign Diseases of the Liver and the Digestive Carcinology

Chapter 5

Hydatid Cysts of the Liver – Diagnosis, Complications and Treatment

Fethi Derbel, Mohamed Ben Mabrouk,
Mehdi Ben Hadj Hamida, Jaafar Mazhoud,
Sabri Youssef, Ali Ben Ali, Hela Jemni, Nadia Mama,
Hasni Ibtissem, Arifa Nadia, Chedia El Ouni,
Walid Naija, Moncef Mokni and Ridha Ben Hadj Hamida

Additional information is available at the end of the chapter

http://dx.doi.org/10.5772/48433

1. Introduction

Hydatid disease in people is mainly caused by infection with the larval stage of the dog tapeworm *Echinococcus granulosus*. It is an important pathogenic, zoonotic and parasitic infection (acquired from animals) of humans, following ingestion of tapeworm eggs excreted in the faeces of infected dogs. Hydatid disease is a major endemic health problem in certain areas of the world [1-3].

Cystic hydatid disease usually affects the liver (50–70%) and less frequently the lung, the spleen, the kidney, the bones, and the brain [1-3]. Liver hydatidosis can cause dissemination or anaphylaxis after a cyst ruptures into the peritoneum or biliary tract. Infection of the cyst can facilitate the development of liver abscesses and mechanic local complications, such as mass effect on bile ducts and vessels that can induce cholestasis, portal hypertension, and Budd-Chiari syndrome [4].

Treatment of hydatid liver cyst has to be considered mandatory in symptomatic cysts and recommended in viable cysts because of the risk of severe complications [1]. The modern treatment of hydatid cyst of the liver varies from surgical intervention to percutaneous drainage or medical therapy. Surgery is still the treatment of choice and can be performed by the conventional or laparoscopic approach. However, laparoscopic approach leads to an important rate of recurrence of the disease. Percutaneous Aspiration-Injection-Reaspiration Drainage (PAIR) seems to be a better alternative to surgery in selected cases.

2. Epidemiology

Echinococcus granulosus is spread almost all over t he world, especially in areas where sheep are raised, and is endemic in Asia, North Africa, South and Central America, North America, Canada and the Mediterranean region. In many countries, hydatid disease is more prevalent in rural areas where there is a closer contact between people and dogs and various domestic animals which act as intermediate vectors. Hydatid disease remains frequent and endemic in Tunisia [5]

2.1. Life cycle of *Echinococcus granulosus*

The life cycle of E. granulosus requires both an intermediate host usually(a sheep, a cattle, or a swine), and a primary canine host. A man becomes both an accidental and an intermediate host through contact with infected dogs or by ingesting food or water contaminated with eggs of the parasite. One can never be surprised to find out that this disease is most commonly found in the temperate and sheep-raising areas of the world [3]

Once the eggs are ingested, they release larvae into the duodenum. The larvae migrate through the intestinal mucosa and gain access to mesenteric vessels which carry them to the liver. The liver is the site of up to 70% of echinococcal lesions. Larvae that escape hepatic filtering are carried to the lung, the site of an additional 15-30% of lesions. From the lungs, larvae may be disseminated to any part of the body. (figure 1). Larvae that escape the host's defenses and persist in a host organ develop into small cysts surrounded by a fibrous capsule. These cysts grow at a rate of 1-3 cm/year and may remain undetected for years.Thus; they can reach very large sizes before they become clinically evident. The cyst wall contains an outer chitinous layer and an inner germinal layer. The germinal layer may develop internal protrusions and eventually form daughter cysts within the original cyst.

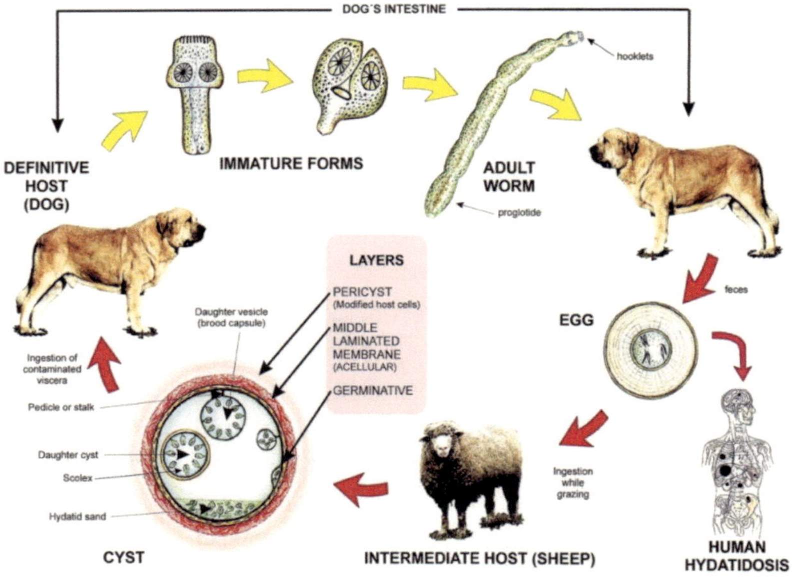

Figure 1. The Life cycle of Echinococcus granulosus.[in 3]

3. Pathology - Hydatid cyst structure

A primary cyst in the liver is composed of three layers: (figure 2)

1. Adventitia (pericyst): consisting of compressed liver parenchyma and fibrous tissue induced by the expanding parasitic cyst.

2. Laminated membrane (ectocyst): is elastic white covering, easily separable from the adventitia. (Figure3-4)

3. Germinal epithelium (endocyst) – is a single layer of cells lining the inner aspects of the cyst and is the only living component, being responsible for the formation of the other layers as well as the hydatid fluid and brood capsules within the cyst. In some primary cysts, laminated membranes may eventually disintegrate and the brood capsules are freed and grow into daughter cysts. Sometimes the germinal Epithelium daughter cysts, which if left untreated may cause recurrence.

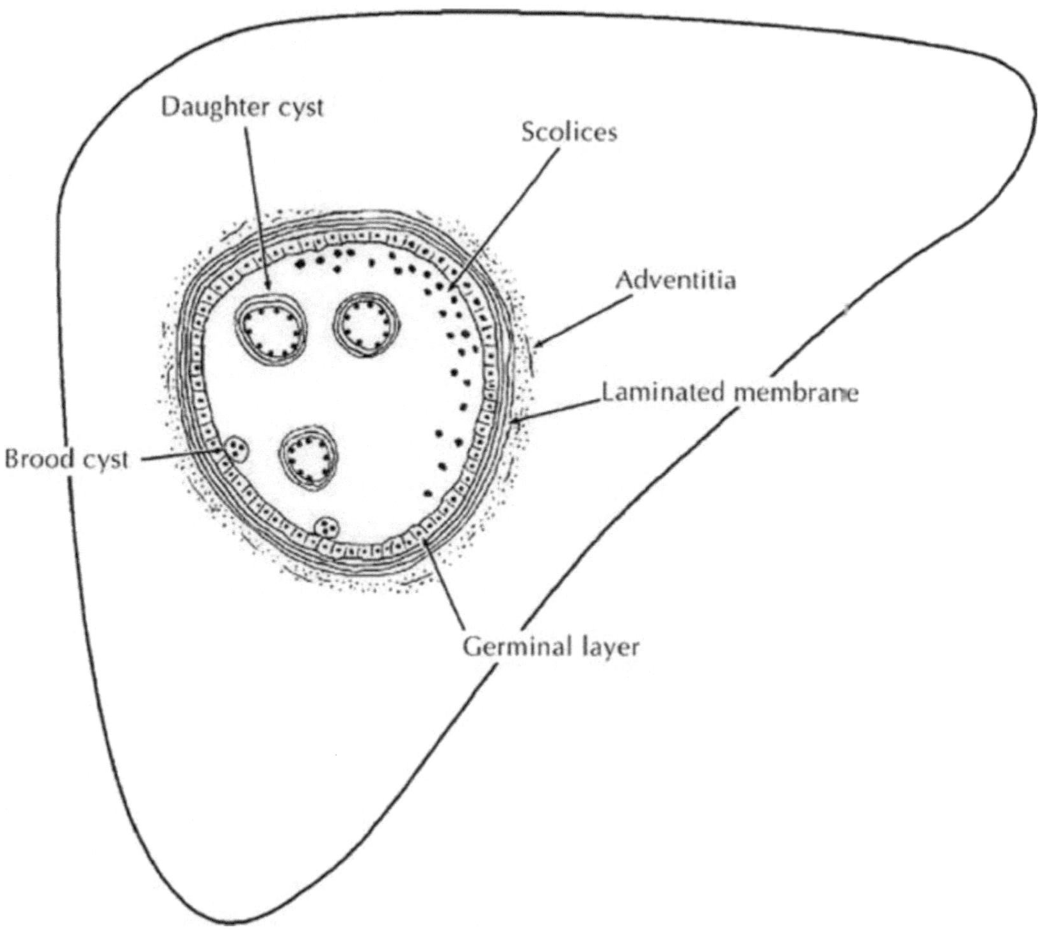

Figure 2. Hydatid cyst of the liver

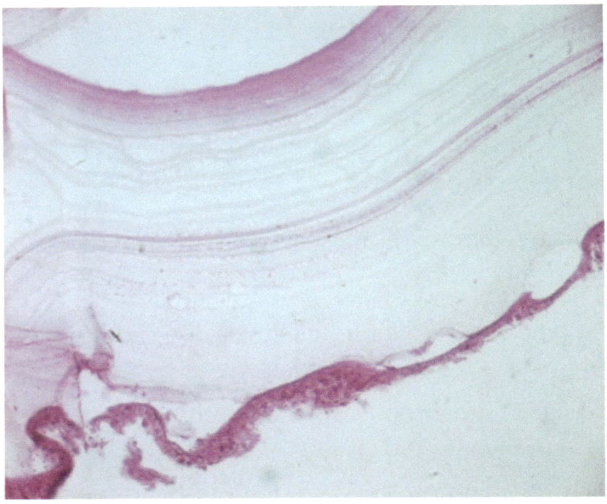

Figure 3. Cystic structures with laminating fibrous wall and inner germinal layer

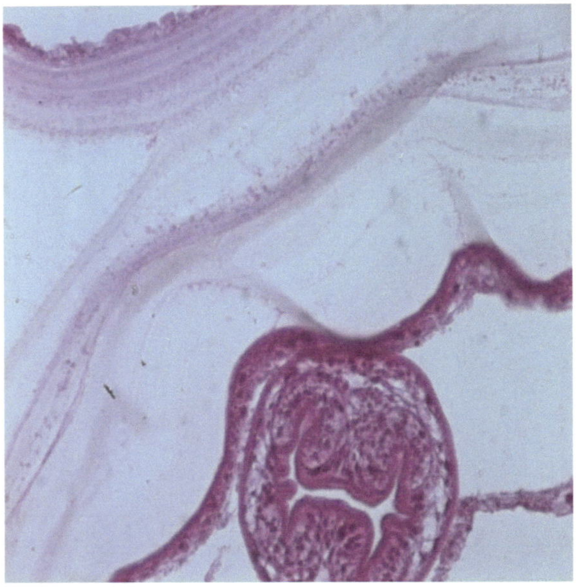

Figure 4. Tissue section of a hydatid cyst showing daughter cyst

4. Natural history and genesis of complications:

Natural history of the hydatid cyst can be divided into two phases:

- The first phase is that of growth during which rupture can occur when the pressure of the hydatid liquid becomes more important than resistance of the hydatic wall (pericyst). Finally, the complications such as acute allergic manifestations, infection, jaundice, vomique, are only the consequence of the rupture of the cystic wall.
- The second phase is a phase of ageing and of progressive involution. It is the consequence of the overproduction of scolices and daughter cysts. During this phase,

the hydatid cyst will be full of scolices and membranes which replace the hydatic liquid. Calcifications occur in the pericyst; the host is at the origin of the image of pericystic wall. Then the reaction of the host leads to a progressive calcification of the walls.

The hydatid cyst is unique and localized in the right lobe of the liver in 65%. The most frequent extrahepatic locations are the lungs, the spleen and the peritoneum. Liver (55–70%) is the obvious first site after entry through the gut and passage in the portal circulation. Most cysts tend to be located in the right lobe. As the cysts enlarge local pressure causes a mass effect on surrounding tissue producing commensurate symptoms and signs. These may be generalized with upper abdominal pain and discomfort or more specific. Such as; obstructive jaundice. Biliary rupture may occur through a small fissure or bile duct fistula. A wide perforation allows the access of hydatid membranes to the main biliary ducts, which can cause symptoms simulating choledocholithiasis. Alternatively, it may produce a picture very similar to ascending cholangitis with fever, pain and jaundice.

5. Complications of hydatid cyst of the liver:

Echinococcal cysts of the liver can cause complications in about 40% of cases. The most common complications in order of frequency are infection, rupture to the biliary tree; rupture to the peritoneal cavity; rupture to the pleural cavity.

However, rupture in the gastrointestinal tract; bladder and the vessels are very rare.

5.1. Infection

It is the most common complication and can be somewhat symptomatic. The evolution of an infected hydatid cyst is usually latent, subacute and is clinically translated by pains in the right hypochondrium, hepatomegaly, and fever [1-3].

5.2. Intrabiliary rupture of hydatid cyst

Intrabiliary rupture of a hepatic hydatid cyst is a common complication and may occur in 2 forms: an occult rupture, in which only the cystic fluid drains to the biliary tree and is observed in 10-37% of the patients; and frank rupture, which has an overt passage of intracystic material to the biliary tract and is observed in 3-17% of the patients. Intrabiliary rupture mainly occurs in centrally localized cysts, and an intracystic water pressure up to 80 cm is also a predisposing factor for the rupture. Intrabiliary rupture occurs in the right hepatic duct (55-60% cases), left hepatic duct (25-30% cases), hepatic duct junction, common bile duct (CBD), or cystic duct (8-11%); perforation into the gallbladder may be observed in 5-6% of cases.

The incidence of rupture into the biliary tree ranges between 3 and 17% [4-6].

The rupture of the hydatid cyst in the biliary ducts and the migration of the hydatid material in the biliary tree lead to the apparition of other biliary complications like: cholangitis, sclerosis odditis, hydatid biliary lithiasis etc.

When ruptured into biliary tree, hydatid cysts commonly manifest with findings of biliary obstruction and cholangitis. Diagnosis of this complication can usually be made by using ultrasound and abdominal CT scan.

The presence of dilated common bile duct, jaundice, or both in addition to a cystic lesion of liver and bile ducts dilatation at CT-scan is strongly suggestive of a hydatid cyst with intrabiliary rupture. (Figure 5)

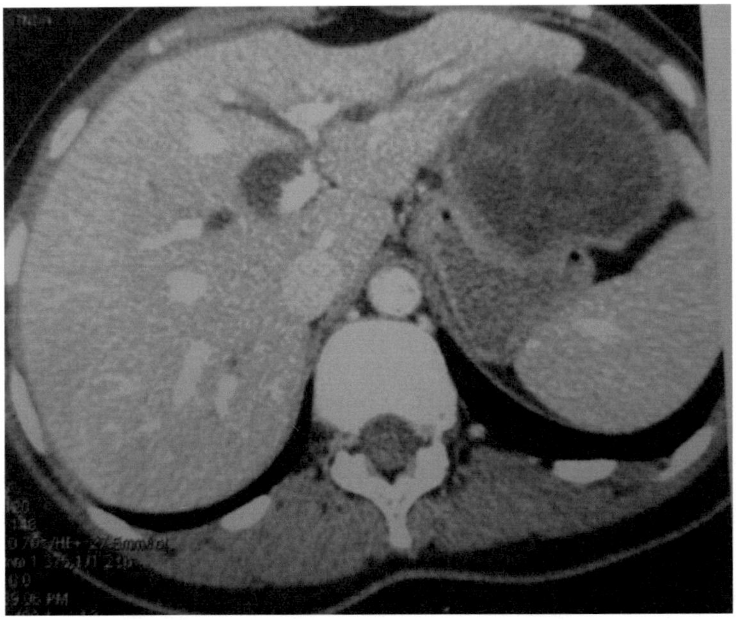

Figure 5. CT scan showing hepatic hydatid cyst with dilatation of left intra hepatic duct

5.3. The rupture in the thorax

Thoracic complications of hepatic hydatid cysts result from the proximity of hydatid cysts in the liver and the diaphragm and are seen in approximately 0.6% to 16% of cases.

Several factors, such as pressure gradient between thoracic and abdominal cavities, mechanical compression and ischemia of the diaphragm, sepsis in the hepatic cyst, or chemical erosion by bile, participate in promoting Intrathoracic evolution of hydatid cysts of the hepatic dome.[6-10]

Intrathoracic rupture of hepatic hydatid cyst is a rare but a severe condition causing a spectrum of lesions to the pleura, lung parenchyma, and bronchi. Cyst erosion is associated with pericystic inflammation. Adhesion formation determines whether the rupture is confined to lung parenchyma or the free pleural space, or both. Bronchobiliary fistula leads to hemoptysis and cyst expectoration.

The clinical presentation is predominately pulmonary, with abdominal symptoms being less frequent [11-12].Coughs, expectoration, and dyspnea are present in 30% of cases.

Diagnosis of thoracic complications is performed with Thoraco-abdominal CT-scan which shows the liver hydatid cyst, and the thoracic complication and sometimes could show the diaphragmatic fistula(figure 6-8). The treatment of this complication is usually made through abdominal approach associated to percutaneous drainage of the pleural collection. The indications for thoracotomy become rare.

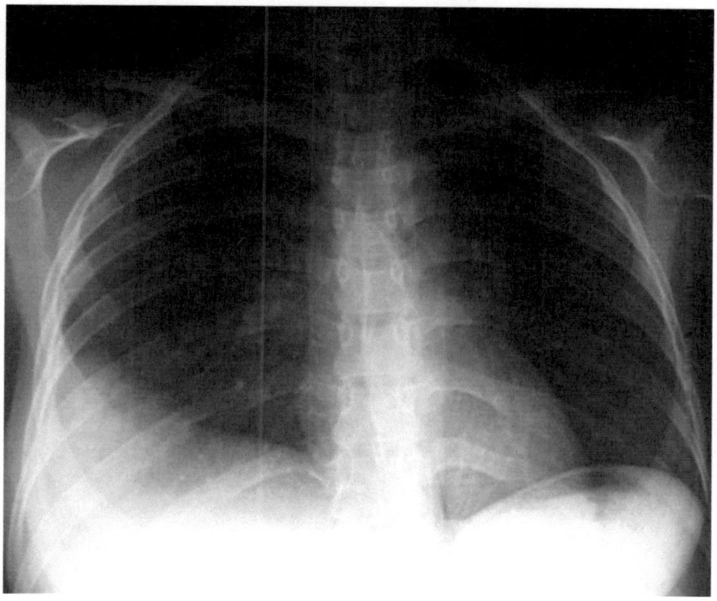

Figure 6. Chest radiograph showing a right pleural effusion with atelectasis

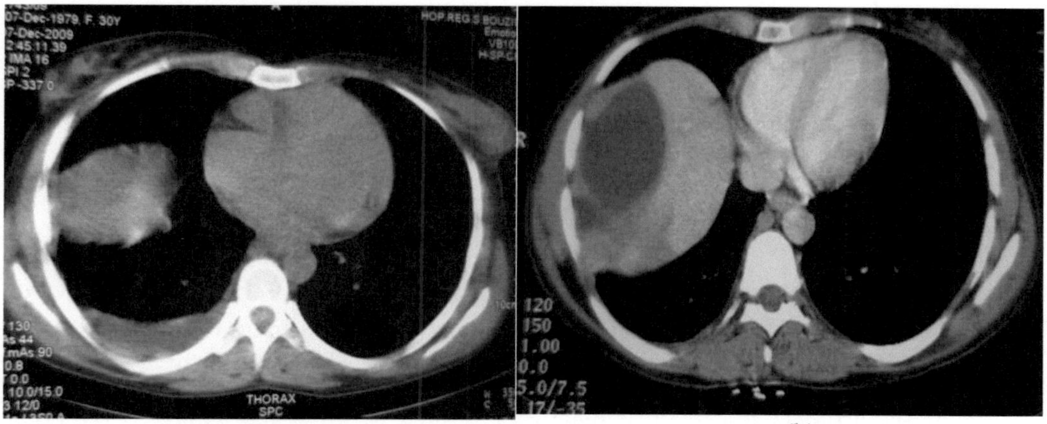

(a) (b)

Figure 7. Thoracic CT-scan showing an atelectasis of the lower lobe of right lung (A) and hydatid cyst of the hepatic dome(B)

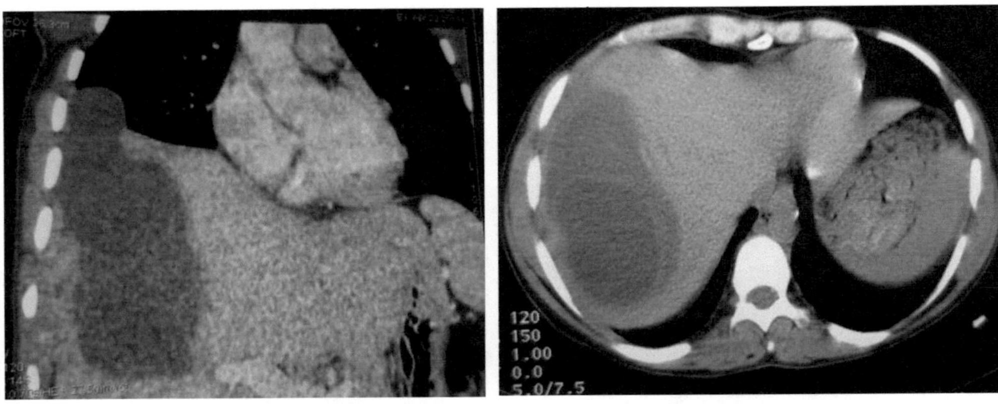

Figure 8. Abdominal CT-scan showing a hepatic hydatid cyst of segment VII with communication with the right pleura

5.4. The rupture in the peritoneum

Rupture of the cyst in the peritoneal cavity is rare and generally followed by anaphylactic reactions.A free intraperitoneal rupture has been reported between 1% and 8% in the literature [13-14].

Intraperitoneal cysts may rupture spontaneously, due to increased intracystic pressure, or as a consequence of trauma [8-9], leading to the spread of hydatid fluid in the intraperitoneal cavity.

Significant risk factors for hydatid cyst perforation include younger age, cyst diameter of >10 cm, and superficial cyst location.

Rupture into the peritoneum may present as acute abdominal pain. Antigenic fluid released into the peritoneal cavity and absorbed into the circulation may present with acute allergic manifestations. Abdominal pain, nausea, vomiting and urticaria are the most common symptoms. Allergic reactions may be seen in 25% of the cases.

In some cases, if the hydatid cyst contains bile due to associated rupture in the biliary tree, the patient will present peritonitis or even of hydatid choleperitonitis.

If the rupture is insidious, the release of brood capsules, scolices and even daughter cysts from a ruptured hydatid cyst into the peritoneal cavity leads to multiple cysts in the peritoneal cavity. This phenomenon is called secondary echinococcosis [15-16]. (Figure 9-13)

The diagnosis of this complication is mainly performed with the abdominal CT-scan that shows the hydatid cyst of the liver generally collapsed and peritoneal effusion or daughter cysts. In secondary echinococcosis, the CT –scan shows the hydatid cysts and many peritoneal cysts.

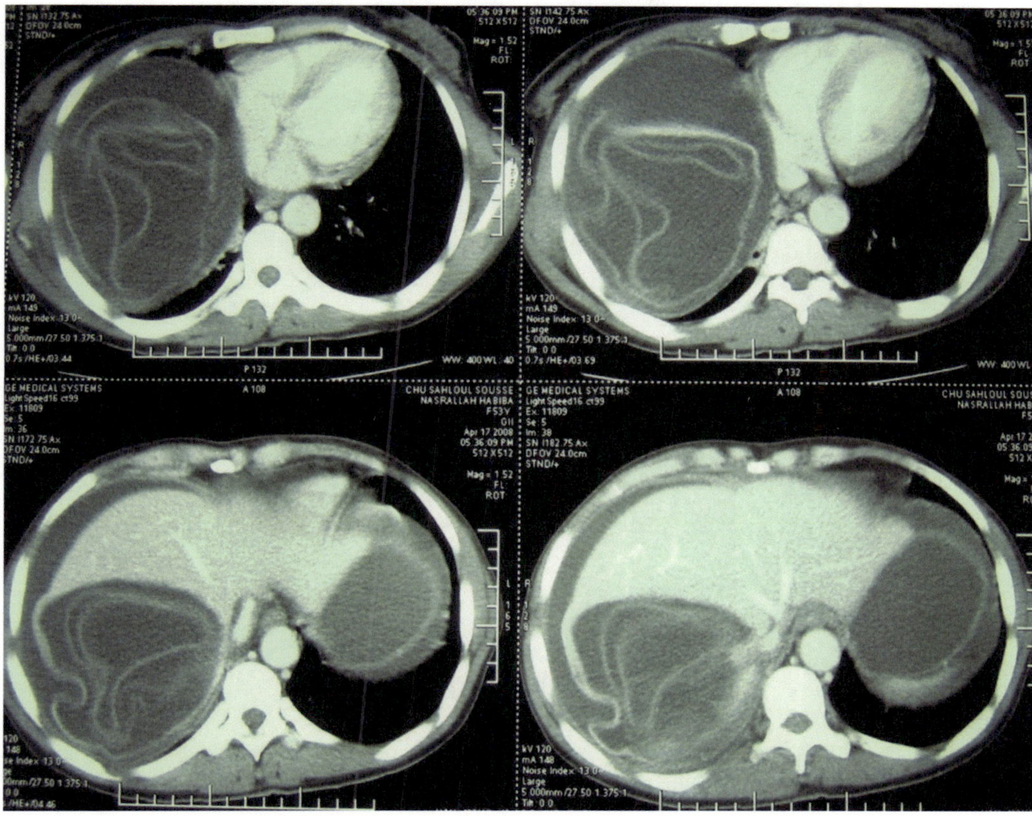

Figure 9. CT scan showing a rupture hydatid cyst of the liver in the peritoneum

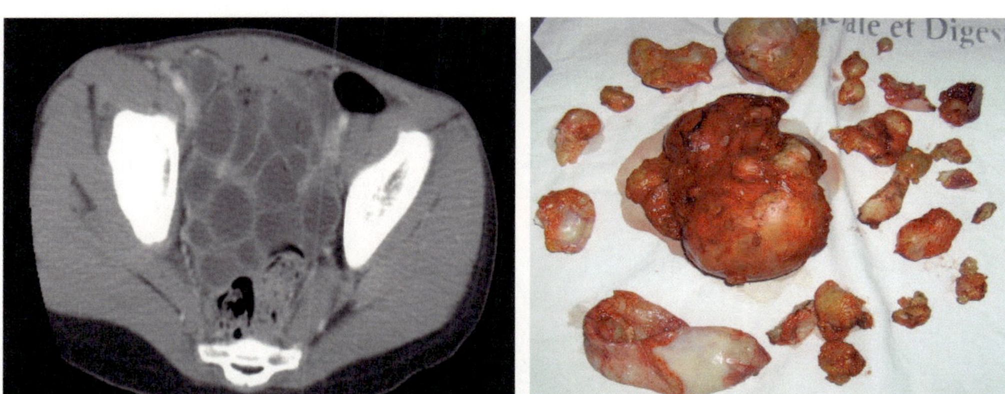

(a) (b)

Figure 10. CT-scan of the abdomen showing multiple hydatid cysts in the peritoneal cavity due to rupture of hepatic hydatid cyst (secondary echinococcosis)(A). Multiple peritoneal cysts(B)

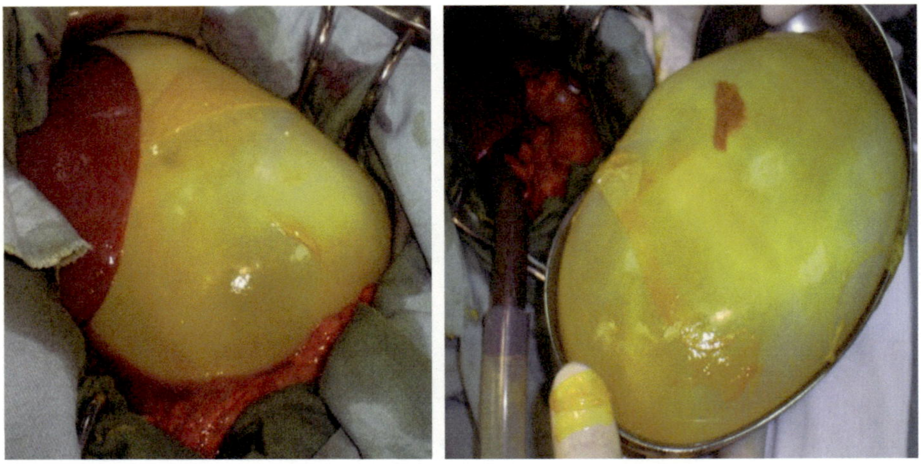

Figure 11. An operative view in a 12 years old male showing a hydatid cyst of the liver with spontaneous rupture in peritoneum

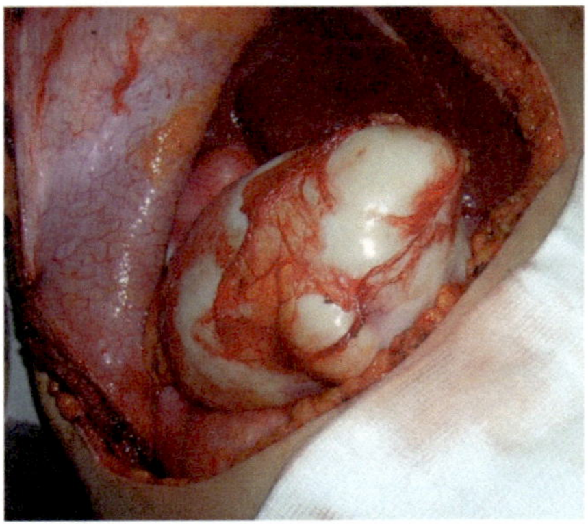

Figure 12. Operative view showing a hydatid cyst of the peritoneum

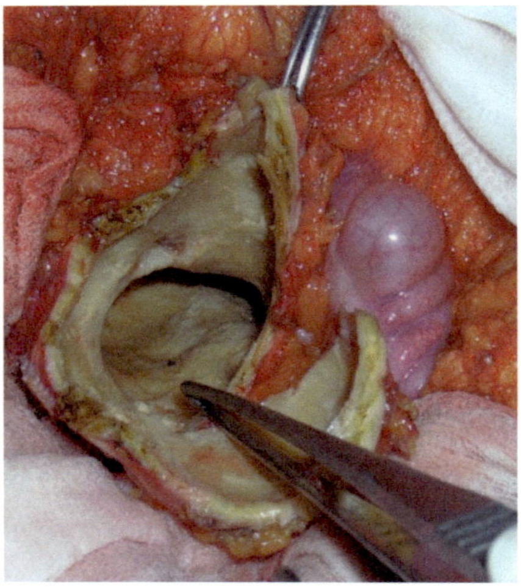

Figure 13. Operative view showing a peritoneal echinococcosis

5.5. Other complications

Some complications of the hydatid cyst of the liver are very rare.

About fistulization to the skin, It occurs most often by a cutaneous orifice leaving pus welling and sometimes hydatid membranes [17-18].

Portal hypertension (pre-hepatic, hepatic, post-hepatic) is a very rare complication of hydatid cyst of liver.The compression of the hepatic veins can be responsible for Budd-Chiari syndrome and portal hypertension [19-20]. (fig 14-15)

Vascular erosions are very rare complications of the hydatid cysts of the liver. The vessels could be either the hepatic vein or the veina cava. Some spontaneous ruptures into the veina cava have been described [19].

Acute abdominal pains with a sudden decrease in the volume of cyst and release of daughter vesicles during vomiting (hydatimesis) or in stool (hydatidentery) are highly suggestive of the opening of the cyst in the digestive tract.(fig 16-17)

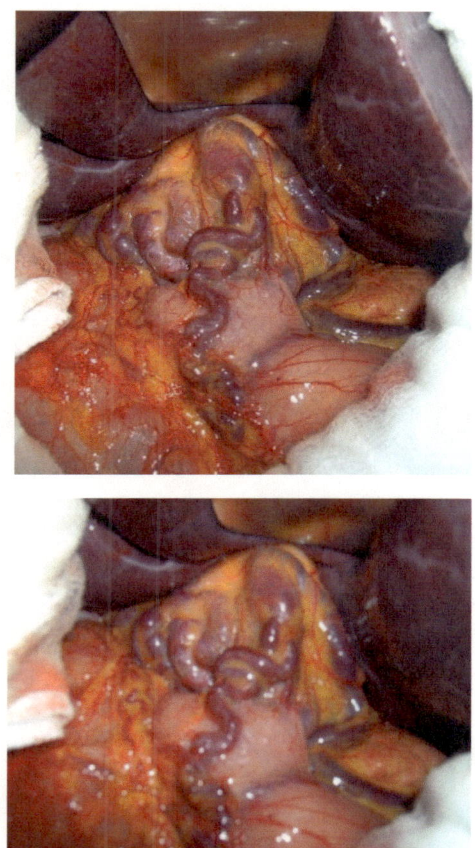

Figure 14. Operative view showing a hydatid cyst of the liver with portal hypertension

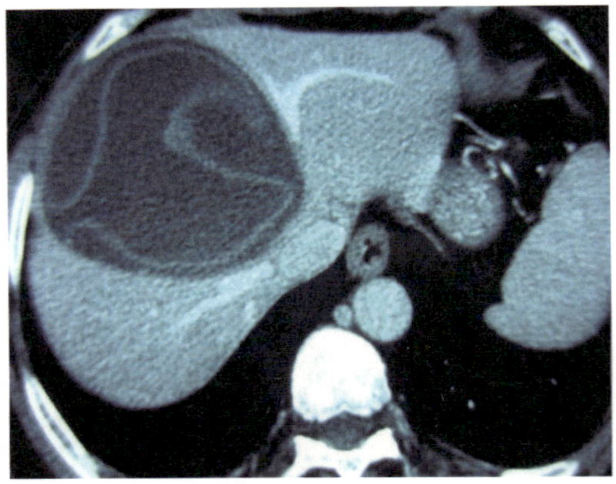

Figure 15. CT scan showing a central hepatic cyst with vascular compression

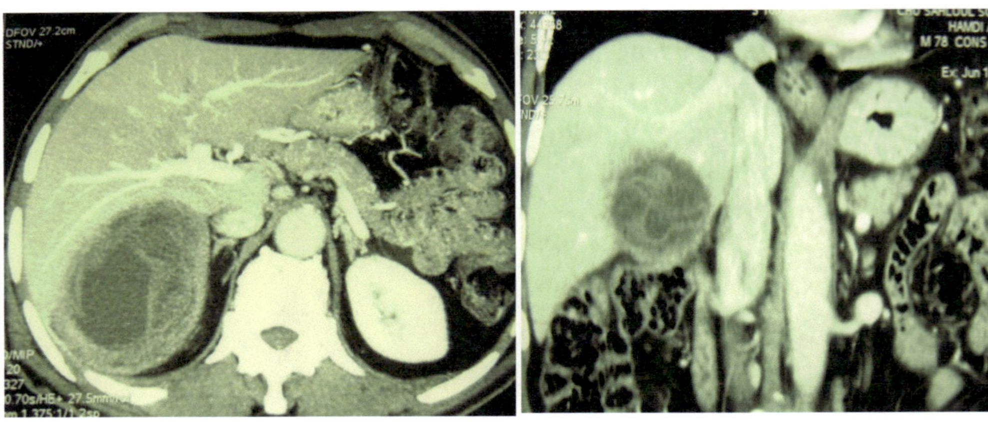

Figure 16. CT-scan : hydatid cyst of the segment V showing a large fistula between the cyst and the right colon

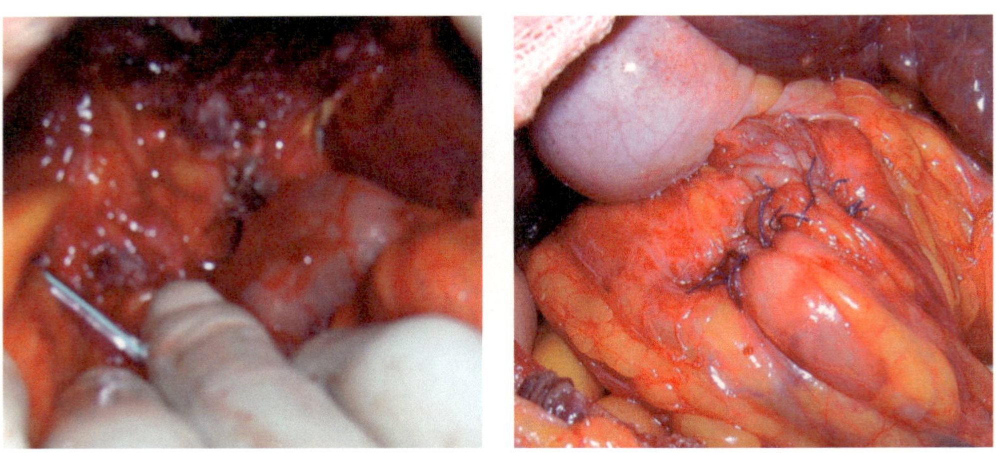

(a) (b)

Figure 17. Operative view showing the colonic fistula (A) and the suture of the fistula after cysto-colonic deconnexion(B)

6. Diagnosis

6.1. Clinical feature

After infection with Echinococcus granulosus, humans are usually asymptomatic for a long time. The growth of the cyst in the liver is variable, ranging from 1 mm to 5 mm in diameter per year. Most primary infections consist of a single cyst, but up to 20%-40% of infected people have multiple cysts. The symptoms depend not only on the size and number of cysts, but also on the mass effect within the organ and upon surrounding structures.[21]

6.1.1. Non complicated cysts

Hydatid cyst of the liver is frequently silent and only diagnosed incidentally during abdominal investigation for other pathology. The clinical signs appear gradually with the increase volume of the cyst. The most common symptom, when it occurs, is right upper quadrant or epigastric pain and the most common findings on examination are an enlarged liver and a palpable mass. Pressure effects are initially vague. They may include non-specific pain, cough, low-grade fever, and the sensation of abdominal fullness. As the mass grows, the symptoms become more specific because the mass impinges on or obstructs specific organs.

6.1.2. Complicated cysts

Patients may also present with complications of the cyst such as biliary communication, intraperitoneal rupture (spontaneous or post-traumatic) and, rarely, intrathoracic or intrapericardial rupture.

Cyst rupture can be associated with anaphylaxis secondary to the highly antigenic content of the cyst fluid or may be silent and present with multiple intraperitoneal cysts.

With secondary infection, tender hepatomegaly, chills, and spiking temperatures occurs. Urticaria and erythema occur in cases of generalized anaphylactic reaction. With biliary rupture the classic triad of jaundice, biliary colic and urticaria occurs.

The diagnosis is most easily set by ultrasound or other imaging techniques such as CT-scan or MRI, combined with case history. Serology tests such as ELISA or immunoblotting can be used in addition, being 80-100% sensitive for liver cysts but only 50-56% for lungs and other organs [21]. False positive reactions may occur in persons with other tapeworm infections, cancer, or chronic immune disorders. Whether the patient has detectable antibodies depend on the physical location, integrity and viability of the cyst. Patients with senescent, calcified or dead cysts usually are sero-negative. Patients with alveolar echinococcosis have most of the time detectable antibodies. Fine needle biopsy should be avoided if dealing with E. granulosus since there is a great danger of leakage with subsequent allergic reactions and secondary recurrence.

A great part of the patients treated for hydatid disease get their diagnosis incidentally, seeking medical care for other reasons.

The time at when a previously silent cyst gives rise to pathology depends both on the size of the cyst, but also on its location, making presenting symptoms of cystic echinococcosis highly variable. Most presenting features are caused by the pressure that the enlarged cyst expels on its surroundings, but may also appear if there is a rupture of a cyst.

Symptoms leading to diagnosis mostly include abdominal pain, jaundice (caused by biliary duct obstruction) or a palpable mass in the hepatic area. Cysts in the liver may also cause cirrhosis.

If the cyst is damaged, there may be a leakage of fluid from inside. This fluid contains antigens that are highly toxic, causing allergic reactions like fever, asthma, urticaria, and eosinophilia and in some cases anaphylactic shock.

6.2. Investigations

Considering that the early stages of infection are usually asymptomatic, the diagnosis of liver hydatid cyst may often be incidental, associated with an abdominal ultrasonography performed for other clinical reasons. In endemic areas, the presence of symptoms suggestive of hydatid liver cyst in a person with a history of exposure to sheep and dogs supports the suspicion of hydatidosis.

The definitive diagnosis of liver echinococcosis requires a combination of imaging, serologic, and immunologic studies.

Routine laboratory tests are rarely abnormal occasionally eosinophilia may be present in the presence of cyst leakage, or may be normal. Serum alkaline phosphatase levels are raised in one third of patients

6.2.1. Serology and immunological tests.

Serological tests detect specific antibodies to the parasite and are the most commonly employed tools to diagnose past and recent infection with E. granulosus. Detection of IgG antibodies implies exposure to the parasite, while in active infection high titers of specific IgM and IgA antibodies are observed. Detection of circulating hydatid antigen in the serum is of use in monitoring after surgery and pharmacotherapy and in prognosis. ELISA is used most commonly, but alternate techniques are counter-immuno-electrophoresis and bacterial co-agglutination.

Elisa techniques have a high sensitivity above 90% and are useful in mass scale screening. The counter-immuno-electrophoresis has the highest specificity (100%) and high sensitivity

(80 – 90%). CASONI TEST has been used most frequently in the past but is at present considered only of historical importance and has largely been abandoned because of low sensitivity.

Tests of humoral immunity are still widely used to confirm the diagnosis. The sensitivity and specificity of any humoral test depends largely on the quality of the antigens utilised.

Antigens can be derived from the whole parasites or organelles, or soluble antigens from cyst fluid. Indirect immunofluorescence assay (IFA) is the most sensitive test (95%) in patients with hepatic CHD.

The sensitivity and specificity of enzyme-linked immunosorbent assay (ELISA) is highly dependent on the method of antigen preparation, and cross-reactions with other helminthic diseases occur if crude antigens are used. Purified fractions may yield high sensitivities (95%) and specificity (100%).[1,3,21]

6.2.2. Imaging techniques

Imaging modalities range from simple to complex and invasive. Ultrasonography (US) is the screening method of choice.

CT scan is an important preoperative diagnostic tool to determine vascular, biliary or extra hepatic extension, to recognize complications, such as rupture and infections, and therefore to assess respectability[22-28]

However, diagnostic tests such as CT and MRI are mandatory in liver hydatidosis because they allow thorough knowledge regarding lesion size, location, and relations to intrahepatic vascular and biliary structures, providing useful information for effective treatment and decrease in post-operative morbidity

The right lobe is the most frequently involved portion of the liver. Imaging findings in hepatic hydatid disease depend on the stage of cyst growth (whether the cyst is unilocular, contains daughter vesicles, contains daughter cysts, is partially calcified, or is completely calcified.

Plain Radiographs

Plain radiographs of the abdomen and chest may reveal a thin rim of calcification delineating a cyst, or an elevated hemi diaphragm. Both signs are non-specific.

Calcification is seen at radiography in 20%–30% of hydatid cysts and usually manifests with a curvilinear or ringlike pattern representing calcification of the pericyst. During the natural evolution toward healing, dense calcification of all components of the cyst takes place. Although the death of the parasite is not necessarily indicated by calcification of the pericyst, it is implied by a complete calcification (Figure 18)

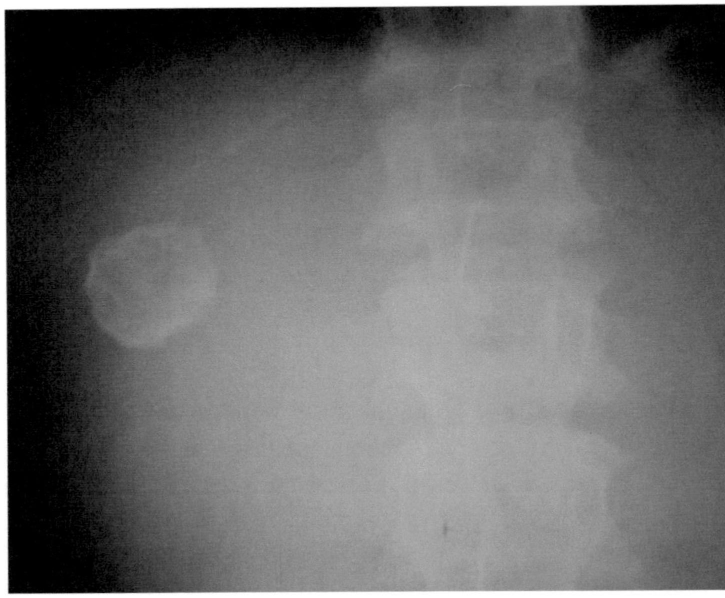

Figure 18. Plain radiograph of the abdomen showing a complete calcification of the cyst

Ultrasonography (US)

Ultrasonography is the screening method of choice. It is currently the primary diagnostic technique and has diagnostic accuracy of 90%. Findings usually seen are:

Solitary Cyst – anechoic univesicular cyst with well defined borders and enhancement of back wall echoes in a manner similar to simple or congenital cysts. Features are suggesting hydatid aetiology include dependent debris (hydatid sand) moving freely with change in position; presence of wall calcification or localized thickening in the wall corresponding to early daughter cysts.

Separation of membranes (ultrasonic water lily sign) due to collapse of germinal layer seen as an undulating linear collection of echoes.

Daughter cysts - probably the most characteristic sign with cysts within a cyst, producing a cartwheel or honeycomb cyst.

Multiple cysts with normal intervening parenchyma (differential diagnosis are necrotic secondaries, Polycystic liver disease, abscess, chronic hematoma and biliary cysts.

Complications may be evident such as echogenic cyst in infection or signs of biliary obstruction (dilated bile ducts with some images corresponding to hyperechoic vesicles or hydatid membranes within the biliary tract) usually implying a biliary communication.

Doppler ultrasonography is indicated to show the reports of hydatid cyst with vascular axes (portal vein, hepatic veins, and inferior vena cava).

However, in the types I and IV, we have to consider differential diagnosis.

Gharbi Classification on Ultrasonography features of Hydatid Cyst [23] ,(Figure 19-20)

Type	Ultrasound Appearance
I	Pure fluid Collection
II	Fluid collection with a split wall **(detached membrane)**
III	Fluid collection with septa **and/or daughter cysts**
IV	Heterogeneous echo pattern **(Hyperechoic with high internal echoes)**
V	Reflecting walls (Cyst with reflecting calcified thick wall)

Type V cysts determined by ultrasound to be calcified and have been assumed to be dead cysts and do not require surgery.

Intra-operative Ultrasonography is an important investigation during surgery for hydatid cyst of the liver.

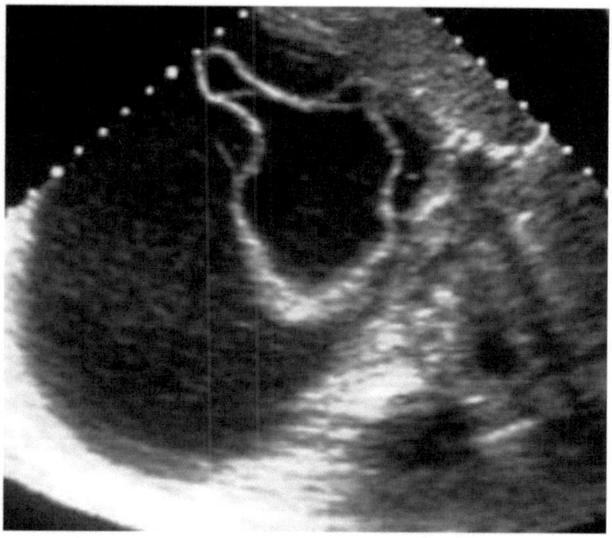

Figure 19. Ultrasonography of Hydatid cyst of the liver type II (Gharbi)

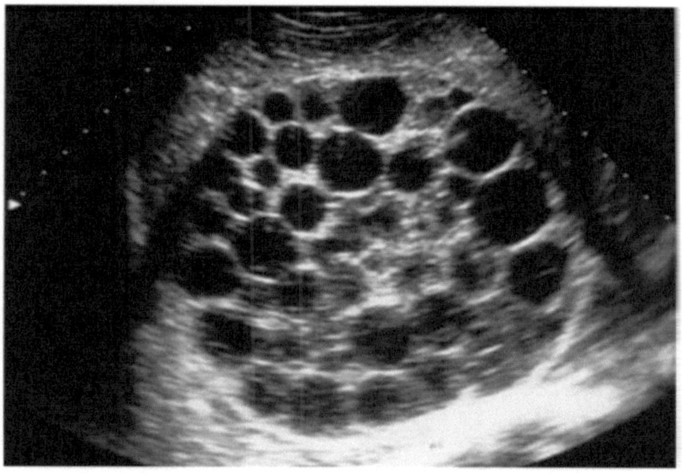

Figure 20. Ultrasonography of Hydatid cyst of the liver Type III (Gharbi)

Different classifications of Ultrasonography have been described in the literature [24-25].

WHO introduced a standardized classification of Ultrasonography images of cystic echinococcosis, to obtain comparable results in patients worldwide and to link disease status with each morphological type of Hydatid cysts (Table 1).

CL Active; Single cysts. Cysts are developing and are fertile. Cyst wall not visible.
CE1 Active; simple cyst often full of hydatid sand (snow flake sign). Visible cyst wall. Fertile.
CE2 Active; multiple, or multi loculated cysts. May appear honeycomb like with daughter cysts. Fertile.
CE3 Transition; degenerating cysts but still contain viable protoscoleces. Often see floating membranes in fluid filled cysts
CE4 Inactive; degeneration is advanced. Cysts may be calcified. Not likely to be fertile. Heterogeneous appearance with few or no daughter cysts.
CE5 Inactive. **Often calcified. Usually infertile.**

(Modified from the WHO classification). Ref www.who.int/emc-documents/zoonoses/docs/whocdscsraph20016.pdf.

Table 1. Classification of hydatid cysts based on the ultrasound appearance.[in 24]

Computed Tomographic scan

Multi detector row computed tomography has the highest sensitivity of imaging of the cyst (100%). It is the best mode to detect the number, size, and location, of the cysts. It may provide clues to presence of complications such as infection, and intrabiliary ruptures. CT features include sharply marginated single or multiple rounded cysts of fluid density (3 – 30 Hounsfield units) with a thin dense rim. [26-28]

It is also helpful in identifying exogenous cysts, and the volume of the cyst can be estimated. CT is an important investigation when there is a diagnostic uncertainty on ultrasound (Type I and IV of Gharbi), when planning surgical intervention or when recurrent disease is diagnosed. In case of peritoneal hydatidosis, CT scan is indicated before surgery to assess the number and the exact localisations of the cysts. (Figure 21-24)

In case of ruptures in the thorax, the CT-scan allows a better study of the lung parenchyma and ensures a percutaneous drainage of the pleural collection.

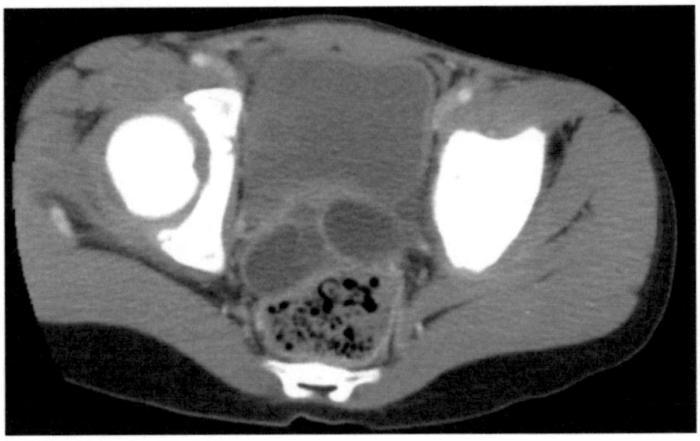

Figure 21. Scan showing a peritoneal hydatidosis

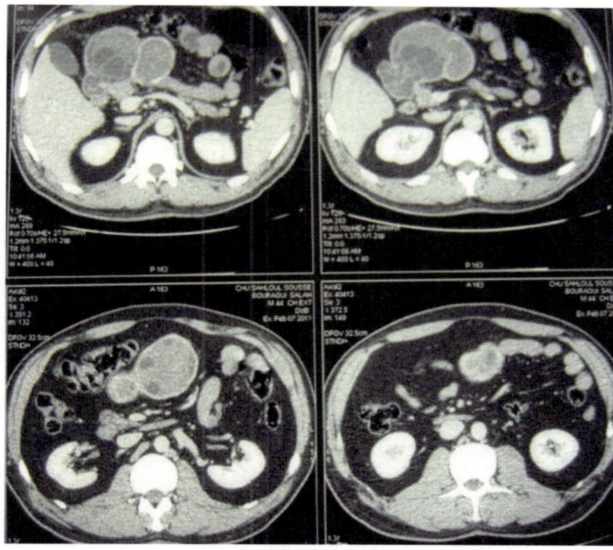

Figure 22. CT- scan of the abdomen showing multiple intra peritoneal hydatid cysts

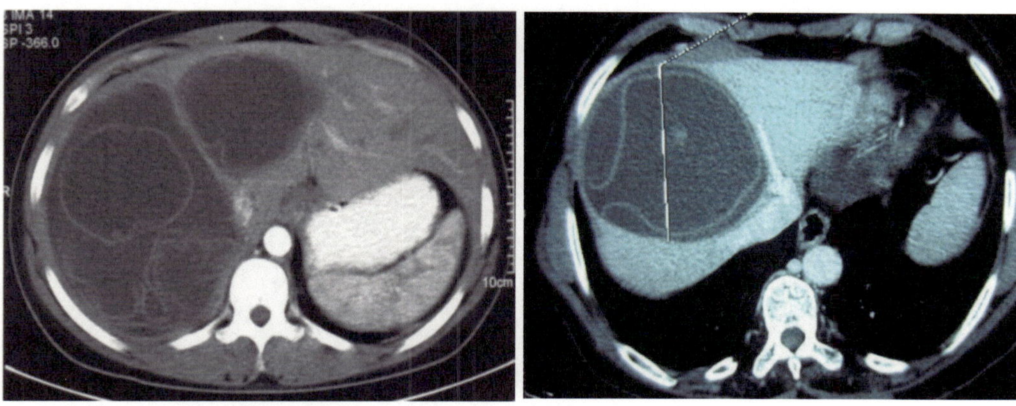

Figure 23. Scan showing typical type II cyst in right lobe of liver.

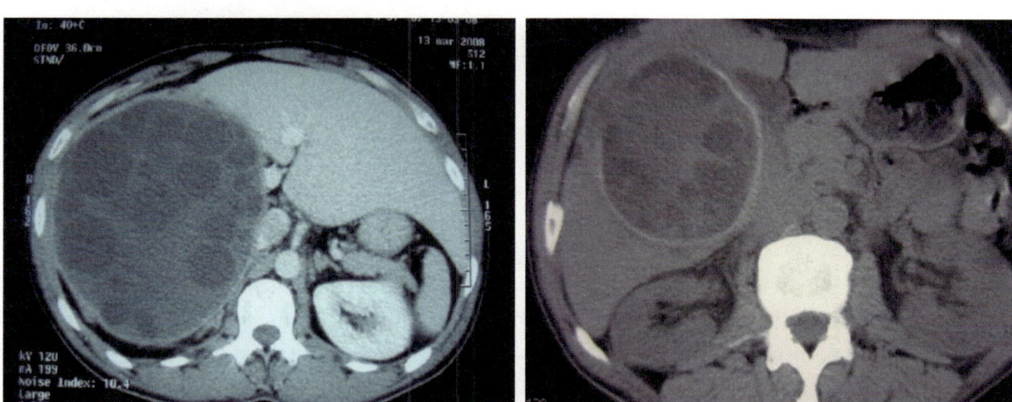

Figure 24. CT scan showing typical type III cyst in right lobe of liver.

Magnetic resonance Imaging (MRI scan) - MRI delineates the cyst capsule better than CT scan, as a low intensity on both T1 and T2 weighted images. However, CT scan is better in demonstrating mural calcifications, cysts less than 3 cm may not show any specific features and small peritoneal cysts may be missed. Magnetic resonance imaging (MRI) adds little to CT scanning. In the routine, this investigation is rarely required as a diagnostic tool for liver hydatidosis.[22,30, 32]

Endoscopic retrograde cholangiopancreatography (ERCP) remains an important tool in cases where a rupture into the biliary tree has occurred, allowing both the diagnosis of major biliary communication and clearance of the common bile duct (CBD) prior to surgery or intervention by the means of sphincterotomy [34]

Direct cholangiography: intra-operative cholangiography is performed through a cystic drain or a T-Tube in a suspected intrabiliary rupture and bile duct obstruction. This method is used to detect post-operative complications following surgery. **(Figure 25)**

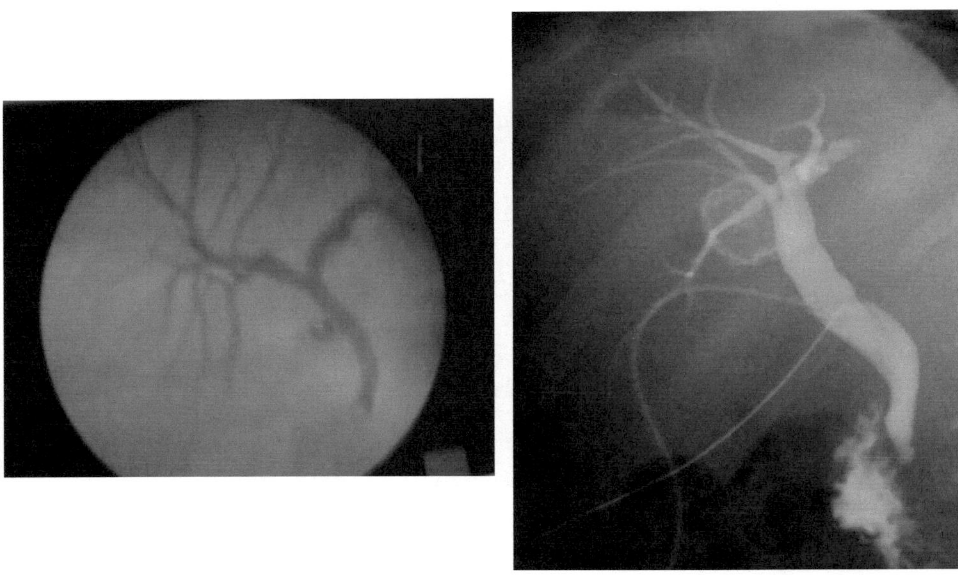

Figure 25. Intra-operative cholangiography showing a daughter cyst in the CBD (A)- post - operative cholangiography (B)

7. Treatment

7.1. General considerations

Surgery remains the gold standard treatment for hydatid liver disease. The aim of surgical intervention is to inactivate the parasite, to evacuate the cyst along with resection of the germinal layer, to prevent peritoneal spillage of scolices and to obliterate the residual cavity. It can be performed successfully in up to 90% of patients if a cyst does not have a risky localisation. However, surgery may be impractical in patients with multiple cysts localised in several organs and if surgical facilities are inadequate. The introduction of chemotherapy and of the PAIR technique (puncture - aspiration - injection - respiration) offers an alternative treatment, especially in inoperable patients and for cases with a high surgical risk. Cysts with homogeneously calcified cyst walls need, probably, no surgery but only a 'wait and observe' approach.

The choice of an optimal treatment should be carefully assessed in each case.[33-34]

The principles of hydatid surgery are

Total removal of all infective components of the cysts;
the avoidance of spillage of cyst contents at time of surgery;
management of communication between cyst and adjacent structures;
management of the residual cavity;
Minimize risks of operation.

All the surgical procedures can be divided into two large groups, a conservative group and a radical one. The conservative technique communication between cyst and adjacent structures;

7.2. The conservative technique

Conservative procedures are safe and technically simple, and are useful in the management of uncomplicated hydatid cysts. Marsupialization was the most common used procedure because it is quick and safe. However, their main disadvantage is the high frequency of postoperative complications, the most common being bile leak from a cyst-biliary communication, bilomas and bile peritonitis (4%-28%).

7.3. Radical surgical procedures

Radical surgical procedures include cystectomy, pericystectomy, lobectomy and hepatectomy. Radical procedures have lower rate of complications and recurrences but many authors consider them inappropriate, claiming that intraoperative risks are too high for a benign disease. [35-39]

a. **Cystectomy** –. The procedure involves removal of hydatid cyst, comprising laminar layer, germinal layer and cyst contents (daughter cysts and brood capsules). The procedure is simple to perform and has low recurrence rates.(Figure 26-29) The management of the residual cavity is a challenging problem especially in patients with giant hydatid Cysts. Various techniques have been described for the management of residual cavities, such as; external drainage, Capitonnage and omentoplasty
b. **Pericystectomy** – this procedure involves a non-anatomical resection of cyst and surrounding compressed liver tissue. This is technically a more difficult procedure than cystectomy and can be associated with considerable blood loss; it can also be hazardous in the case of large and complicated cysts when the cyst distorts vital anatomical structures such as; hepatic veins or biliary ducts. (Figure.30-31)
c. **Hepatic resections** – The arguments against hepatic resection as a primary modality of treatment are :firstly, outside of the dedicated liver units there is considerable

morbidity and mortality from resection of what is essentially a benign condition .What is more, the distortion of the anatomy makes surgery harder.

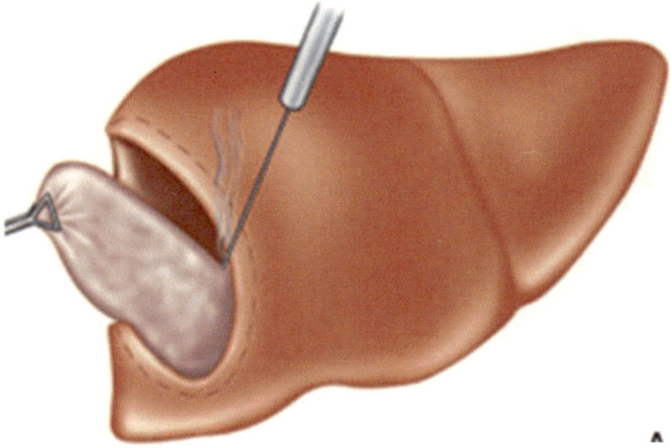

Figure 26. Radical surgery: partial cystectomy [in 55]

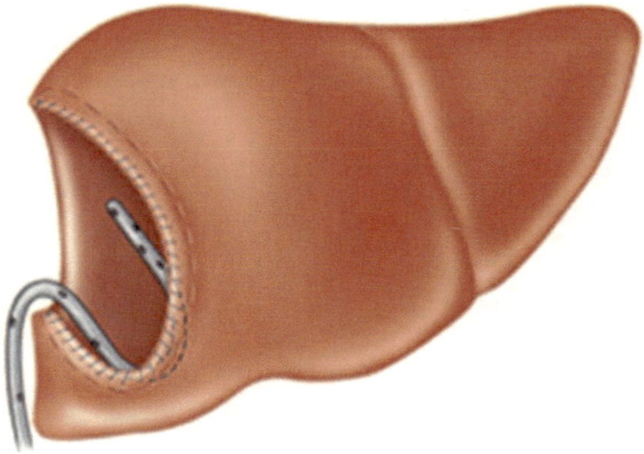

Figure 27. Drainage of the residual cavity after partial cystectomy [in 55]

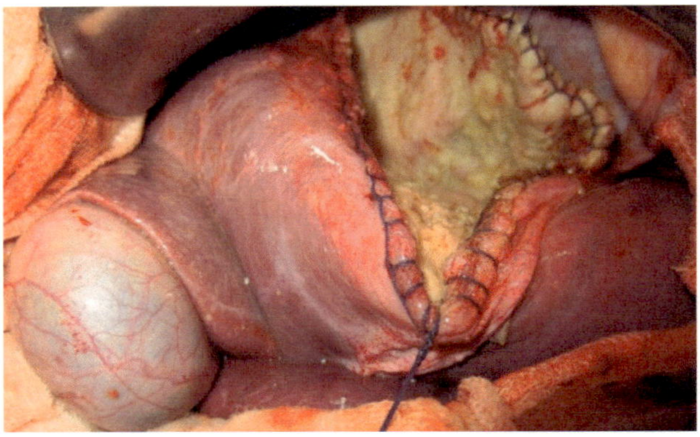

Figure 28. A 34- year- old patient operated for hydatid cyst of segment VIII. Partial cystectomy and capitonnage

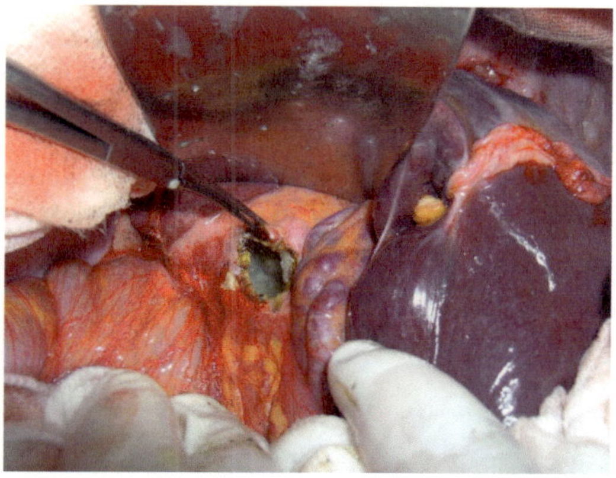

Figure 29. Hydatid cyst of liver with portal hypertension: partial cystectomy

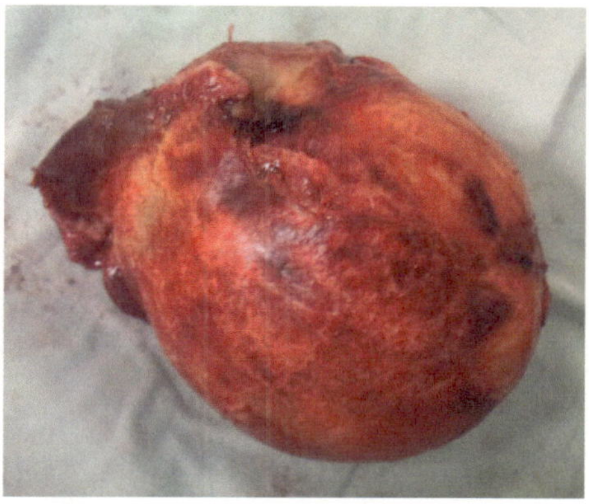

Figure 30. Total pericystectomy for a hydatid cyst the lower surface of the right hepatic lobe.

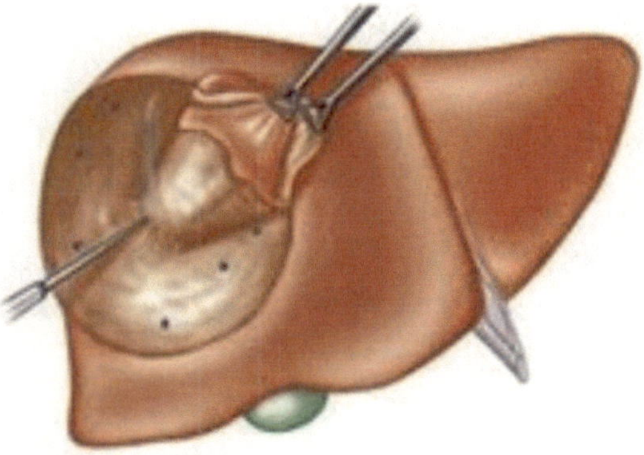

Figure 31. Technique of the pericystectomy in [34]

7.4. Laparoscopic management of hydatid cysts

The rapid development of laparoscopic techniques has encouraged surgeons to replicate principles of conventional hydatid surgery using a minimally invasive approach. Several reports have confirmed the feasibility of laparoscopic hepatic hydatid surgery [40-42]

A special instrument has been developed for the removal of the hydatid cyst with the laparoscope called the perforator-grinder-aspirator apparatus. Different instruments have been described to try to avoid leackage of daughter cysts and scolices.

Laparoscopic has some advantages compared to open surgery. In fact this approach to liver hydatid cyst offers a lower morbidity outcome and a shorter hospital stay and it is also associated with a faster surgery. In addition to that advantage, Laparoscopic procedure gives a better visual control of the cyst cavity under magnification which allows a better detection of biliary fistula. This approach is possible only in selected cases.

The Criteria to exclude laparoscopic treatment of hydatid cyst of liver are

Rupture of the cyst in biliary tract
Central localization of the cyst
Cysts dimension > 15 cm
Number of cysts > 3
Thickened or calcified walls
opening of bile ducts that leak bile

Nevertheless, a disadvantage of laparoscopy is the lack of precautionary measures to prevent spillage under the high intraabdominal pressures caused by pneumoperitoneum, allergic reactions are more common in laparoscopic interventions due to peritoneal spillage, though the length of stay is generally shorter and morbidity rates are lower in comparison with open procedures. [40]

Laparoscopic experience has shown that spillage of scolices-rich cyst fluid or daughter cysts is common, and it is difficult to evacuate the cysts without spillage in the absence of the proven techniques available to open surgery [41-42].

Spillage may lead to peritoneal hydatidosis

7.5. Complications of surgery

1. Morbidity: Biliary leakage is the most frequent postoperative complication following surgery for hydatid cysts of liver. The rate varies between 6% and 28%. Although most of the external biliary fistulas close spontaneously, they may be persistent in 4%-27.5% of the cases.(figure 32)

Endoscopic sphincterotomy is performed after a 3-week waiting period in patients with low-flow fistulas or can be performed earlier in patients with high-flow fistulas [43-45]

Some other complications can occur in the post-operative period such as; infection of the residual cavity; which is mainly true for big hydatid cysts, in the hepatic dome and treated by partial cystectomy. This complication is more frequent when the pericyst is thick and calcified. This complication needs in some cases reoperation or percutaneous drainage under CT-scan guidance. For this reason, some authors recommend this type of cysts, a total pericystectomy.

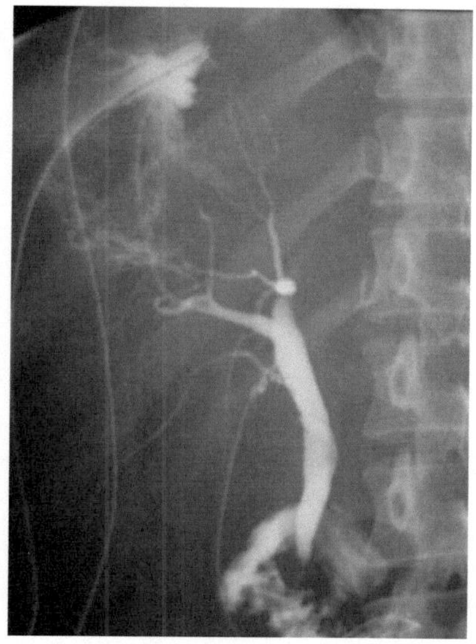

Figure 32. Post-operative cholangiography showing a cysto-biliary fistula

2. Mortality: The surgical management of hydatid disease of liver carries a mortality rate of 0.9 to 3.6 %.
3. Recurrence rate varies with type of surgery; it is estimated up to 11.3 % within 5 years.

7.6. Percutaneous treatment of hydatid cyst

PAIR (puncture, aspiration, injection, and reaspiration) is a percutaneous treatment technique for hydatid disease. This technique was proposed in 1986 by the Tunisian team that first used it in a prospective study [48]. In this minimally invasive method, a needle is introduced into the cyst under ultrasound guidance.

Since that time, its use in the treatment of hydatid cysts has been somewhat controversial [46-50]. However, as this technique has become more common and its safety and efficacy have been reported in the literature [51-56, it has been increasingly accepted as a treatment option for hydatid disease. The World Health Organization currently supports PAIR as an effective alternative to surgery, although its use is limited.

The World Health Organization guidelines for indications and contraindications of PAIR are as follows:[54]

1. Indications for PAIR

Nonechoic lesion greater than or equal to 5 cm in diameter
Cysts with daughter cysts and/or with membrane detachment
Multiple cysts if accessible to puncture
Infected cysts
Patients who refuse surgery.
Patients who relapse after surgery.
Patients in whom surgery is contraindicated

Patients who fail to respond to chemotherapy alone
Children over 3 years.
Pregnant women

2. Contraindications for PAIR
Non cooperative patients
Inaccessible or risky location of the liver cyst
Cyst in spine, brain, and/or heart
Inactive or calcified lesion
Cyst communicating with the biliary tree

Patients should be followed clinically after PAIR treatment. Recurrence is increased in more complicated cysts, including those with multiple daughter cysts.

PAIR should only be performed in highly specialized centers with appropriately trained and experienced staff. In addition, an anaesthesiologist should be present for monitoring and treatment in case of anaphylactic shock. Surgeons should be notified immediately in case of complication.[46-57]

Punctures of hydatid cysts have been discouraged in the past due to the potential risk of Anaphylactic shock and peritoneal dissemination. However, in the recent years percutaneous drainage has been used successfully to treat the hepatic hydatid cysts. Khuroo et al [50] reported 88% disappearance of cysts with percutaneous drainage which was preceded by Albendazole therapy (10 mg/kg body weight) for 8 weeks. In his study, he showed that the efficacy of percutaneous drainage is similar to that of standard treatment with cystectomy, in terms of reducing the size of the cyst and causing its disappearance over a period of up to two years. The advantages of percutaneous drainage include a shorter hospital stay and a lower complication rate.

7.7. Endoscopic management of hydatid cyst

The ERCP is effective in diagnosing biliary tree involvement from the cyst.

The Endoscopic management is useful in presence of intrabiliary rupture, which requires exploration and drainage of the biliary tract and also after surgery in presence of residual hydatid material (membranes and daughter cyst) left in biliary tree. During the endoscopic exploration the biliary tree is cleared of any hydatid material with a balloon catheter or a dormia basket. The endoscopic sphincterotomy is also performed to facilitate drainage of the common bile duct. [44-45]

7.8. Chemotherapy for hydatid disease of liver

Medical treatment of hydatid liver cysts, primarily induced in the 1970's, is based on benzoimidazole carbamates, such as mebendazole and albendazole. It has been proposed that these agents contribute to clinical improvement of the disease by diminishing the size of the cyst. The factors for success seem to be the ability of the drug to penetrate the cyst wall and the persistence of adequate levels of the active metabolites. Albendazole seems to be more effective owing to better penetration and absorption.[58] These agents have actually been used in several studies as a conservative treatment, leading to some decrease or stabilization of the cyst size, especially in cases with small cysts.[58-59] However, their clinical efficacy still remains doubtful. They are used mainly for disseminated systemic disease, inoperable cases, and—combined with surgery—to prevent postoperative recurrence. Side effects of Albendazole therapy are: mild abdominal pain, nausea, vomiting, pruritis, dizziness, alopecia, rash and headaches. Occasionally, leucopoenia, eosinophilia, icterus, and mild elevation in transaminase levels are seen.

The different schedules for the treatment are:

1. Inoperable cases - as primary treatment - 3 cycles
2. Pre-operatively – to reduce the risk of recurrence 6 weeks continuous treatment
3. Post-operatively to prevent recurrence in cases of intraoperative cyst spillage 3 cycles.

In a review by Dziri et al. [60], the authors sought to provide evidence-based answers to the following questions:

- Should chemotherapy be used alone or in association with surgery?
- What is the best surgical technique?
- When are the percutaneous aspiration, injection, and reaspiration technique indicated?

The results showed that chemotherapy is not the ideal treatment for uncomplicated hydatid liver cyst when used alone, and the level of evidence was too low to help in choosing between radical or conservative treatment. Percutaneous drainage plus albendazole proved to be safe and effective in selected patients [38].

7.9. Treatment of hydatid cysts rupture into the biliary tracts

There are two different clinical settings associated with intrabiliary rupture: frank intrabiliary rupture and simple communication. In the former, the cyst content drains to biliary tract and causes cholestatic jaundice. In the latter simple communications are frequently overlooked and could cause post-operative biliary fistulae [37-39]. If the cystobiliary opening was less than 5 mm, spontaneous drainage of the cystic content was uncommon and could be treated by suturing under the direct vision. If the CBD diameter was larger than 5 mm, cystic content migration into the biliary tract would occur in 65% of the cases Vesicles, debris and purulent materials may be found in the biliary ducts. Surgery must be done early. Delay can cause suppurative cholangitis, septicemia and liver abscess formation. The orifice of bile leakage could be seen in 11.7-17.07% of the cases during the operation while this was difficult in posteriorly localized cysts. In these cases, cholangiography could be done by a catheter pushed into the ductus cysticus or the cystobiliary fistula]. The injection of radioopac solution or methylene blue is helpful to diagnose intrabiliary rupture or to see the orifice

Once the Intraoperative cholangiography is performed, biliary communications with the cyst are identified and meticulously sutured. A supraduodenal choledochostomy is made and bile duct cleared by all membranes and debris with the help of choledocoscope. The choledochostomy is closed over a T-tube.

The treatment of the cysto-biliary communication is based on several techniques [5,6, 34, 38].

a. **Direct suture:** small cysto-biliary fistula could be sutured using a resorbable material. This technique could be performed when it is a small fistula
b. **Repair using a T-Tube:**This method allows to restore canal continuity and to drain the hepatic territory of upstream. The T-Tube is kept 4 at 6 weeks and is withdrawn only after cholangiography.
c. **Other techniques:** When a complete pericystectomy is not realizable under good conditions, 2 other techniques of treatment of cysto-biliary communication could be performed:

The transparieto-hepatic fistulization described by Perdromo *et al* [39] which use of a T-tube of which one of the branches is intra-biliary and the other intra-cystic. The T-tube should be kept between 4 and 6 weeks. It could be withdrawn after a cholangiography. (figure 33)

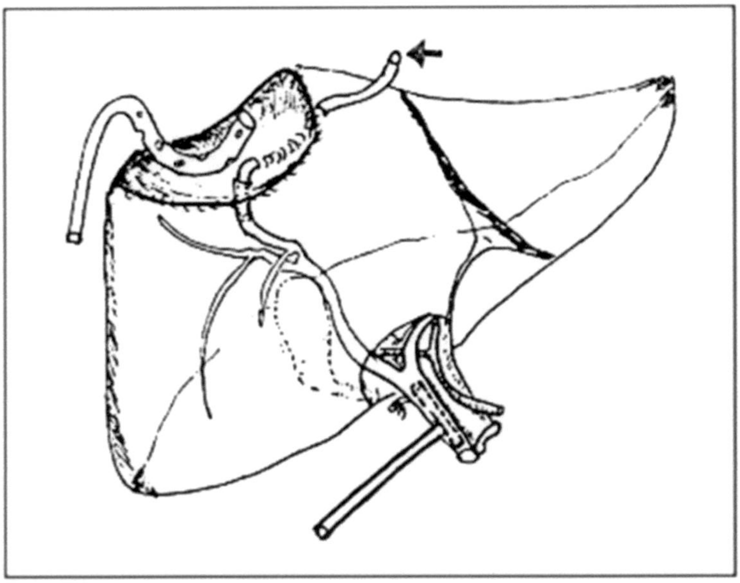

Figure 33. Transparieto-hepatic fistulization (perdromo)

The internal drainage technique described by Goinard (figure 34-35). This technique should be performed for central cyst with a large bilio-cystic fistula. In case of a big hydatid cyst, we should perform a partial pericystectomy to reduce the size of the residual cavity. The pericyst is then sutured and a T-tube is inserted in the common bile duct. This drain should be kept between 5 and 8 weeks, and its withdrawn should be performed after a cholangiography. This technique gives good results in case of central cyst with large cysto-biliary fistula in the right and/or left biliary canal. [6,38,39]

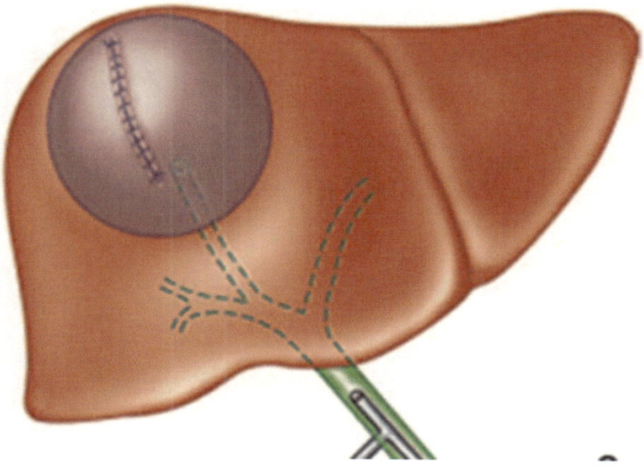

Figure 34. Internal drainage technique [in 34]

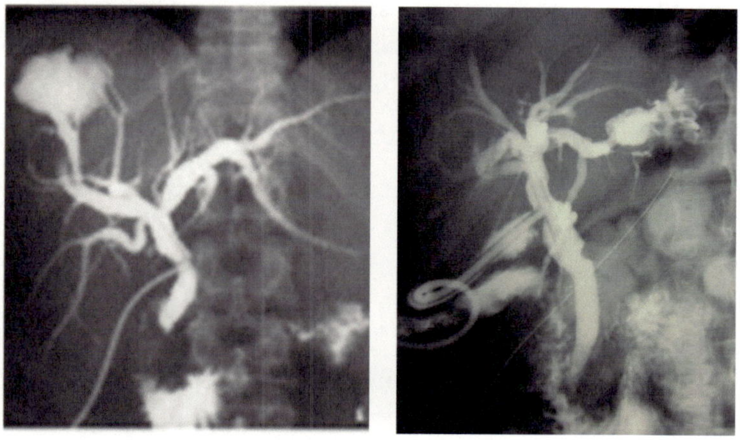

Figure 35. Post-operative cholangiography in a patient treated for hydatid cyst with large bilio-cystic fistula treated with partial cystectomy and internal drainage

8. Conclusion

Hydatid disease remains a continuous public health problem in endemic countries. The liver is the most common site for hydatid disease (75% of cases), followed by the lungs (15%), the spleen (5%), and other organs (5%).

Diagnosis of liver hydatid disease is made with Ultrasonography and computed tomography. Surgery combined with medical treatment by albendazole is effective in the eradication of hepatic hydatid disease and in the prevention of local recurrences.

Although surgery is the recommended treatment for liver hydatid disease, percutaneous treatment has been introduced as an alternative to surgery. PAIR is a valuable alternative to surgery. It is safe and efficient in selected patients

Author details

Fethi Derbel, Mohamed Ben Mabrouk, Mehdi Ben Hadj Hamida, Jaafar Mazhoud, Sabri Youssef, Ali Ben Ali and Ridha Ben Hadj Hamida
Department of Surgery, Sahloul Hospital, Sousse, Tunisia

Hela Jemni, Nadia Mama, Hasni Ibtissem, Arifa Nadia and Chedia El Ouni
Department of Medical Imaging, Sahloul Hospital, Sousse, Tunisia

Walid Naija
Department of Anesthesiology and Intensive Care, Sahloul Hospital, Sousse, Tunisia

Moncef Mokni
Department of Pathology, Farhat Hached Hospital, Sousse, Tunisia

Acknowledgement

We thank Professor Jemni Hela, Ibtissem Hasni and Kalthoum Graiess Tlili for their help in the selection and interpretation of the CT-scan and ultrasound and Dr Jaafar Mazhoud and Dr Mohamed Ben Mabrouk for their great help in collecting the operations view.

A special thank to Mr Bouraoui Chelly for his great help in the critical reading of the manuscript.

9. References

[1] Moro P., Schantz PM. - Echinococcosis: a review- International Journal of Infectious Diseases (2009) 13, 125—133

[2] Nunnari G., Pinzone M R., Gruttadauria S., et al. Hepatic echinococcosis: Clinical and therapeutic aspects. *World J Gastroenterol* 2012; 18(13): 1448-1458

[3] Khanfar N. Hydatid disease: a review and update. Current Anaesthesia & Critical Care (2004) 15, 173–183

[4] Eckert J., Deplazes P. Biological, Epidemiological, and Clinical Aspects of Echinococcosis, a Zoonosis of Increasing Concern. Clin Microbiol Rev. 2004; 17(1): 107–135.

[5] Paksoy M, Karahasanoglu T, Carkman S, Giray S, Senturk H, Ozcelik F, et al. Rupture of the hydatid disease of the liver into the biliary tracts. Dig Surg 1998;15:25–9.

[6] A Zaouche, K Haouet . Management of liver hydatid cysts with a large biliocystic fistula: multicenter retrospective study. Tunisian Surgical Association. World J Surg 2001 Janv, 25(1): 28-39.

[7] Gharbi HA., Mnif J., Ben Abdallah M., Abdelmoula M., Hammou-Jeddi A. Epidemiology of hydatic cyst in Tunisia. Results of investigation by abdominal echography on 3116 inhabitants of Menzel Bourguiba area. Médecine et Maladies Infectieuses- 1986; 16(3): 151–156

[8] Sakhri J., Ben Ali A., Letaief R., Derbel F., Dahmen Y., Ben Hadj Hmida R. Les kystes hydatiques du foie rompus dans le thorax: Aspects diagnostiques et thérapeutiques. J Chir (Paris) 1996;133:437-441

[9] Kilani T., Daoues A., Horchani H., Sellami M. Place de la thoracotomie dans les complications thoraciques des Kystes hydatiques du foie. Ann Chir Thorac Cardiovasc. 1991 ;45 :705-710.

[10] Caporale A., Frittelli P., Della Casa U., et al. Surgical treatment of hydatid cysts of the hepatic dome ruptured into the thoracic cavity. G Chir 1990;11:23-28

[11] Bel Haj Salah R. , Triki W., Bourguiba MB., Ben Moussa M., Zaouche A. Rupture aiguë d'un kyste hydatique foie dans la plèvre droite À propos de deux observations. Chirurgie thoracique et cardiovasculaire - 2011 ; 15(3) : 182-184

[12] Sakhri J, Letaief R, Ben ali A, Derbel F, Ben Hadj Hmida R. Les kystes hydatiques du foie rompus dans le thorax : Quelle voie d'abord choisir ? Ann Chir 1996;50: 284.

[13] Larbi N, Hedfi S, Selmi M, Ben Salah K. La rupture aigue du kyste hydatique du foie dans le péritoine. Ann Chir 2002 ;127:487-488

[14] Kemal Karakaya. Spontaneous rupture of a hepatic hydatid cyst into the peritoneum causing only mild abdominal pain: A case report. World J Gastroenterol February 7, 2007; 13(5)

[15] Anadi Nath Acharya, Shahana Gupta. Peritoneal hydatidosis: A review of seven cases. *Tropical Gastroenterology 2009;30(1):32–34*

[16] İlhan Çiftçi, Hüseyin Yılmaz. Hepatic Hydatid Cyst and Intraperitoneal Free Hydatid Cyst. *Eur J Gen Med 2012;9 (Suppl 1):50-52*

[17] Khila M, Allegue M, Abdesslam M et al. Fistule cutanéo-kysto-bronchique spontanée d'origine hydatique. Tunisie Med 1987; 65:267-270.

[18] H. Bedioui et al. *Kyste hydatique du foie rompu dans la paroi abdominale : A propos d'une observation rare. Med Trop* 2006; 66 : 488-490

[19] Khila M, Said R, Katar S et al. La rupture peropératoire spontanée de la veine cave inférieure dans un kyste hydatique du foie. Tunisie Med 1985;63:399-402.

[20] Ali Emre, Orhan Arioğul, Aydin Alper, Attilâ Ökten, Ali Uras, andSüleyman Yalçin . Hydatid Cysts of Liver and Portal Hypertension- HPB Surgery 1990; 2: 129-133

[21] Wenbao Zhang, Jun Li, Donald P.Mc Manus. Concepts in Immunology and Diagnosis of Hydatid Disease. Clinical Microbiology Reviews, 2003,16(1) :18-36,

[22] Marrone G., Crino F., Caruso S., Mamone G, et al Multidisciplinary imaging of liver hydatidosis. *World J Gastroenterol* 2012; 18(13): 1438-1447

[23] Gharbi H.A., Hassine W., Brauner M.W., Dupuch K. Ultrasound examination of the hydatic liver. *Radiology*, 1981, 139, 459-463

[24] WHO Inform working group on Echinococcosis. International classification of ultrasound images in cystic echinococcosis for application in clinical and field epidemiological settings. Acta Trop 2003; 85(2): 253–61.

[25] Caremani M, Lapini L, Caremani D, Occhini U. Sonographic diagnosis of hydatidosis: the sign of the cyst wall. Eur J Ultrasound 2003;16(3):217–23.

[26] Torricelli P, Martinelli C, Biagini R, Ruggieri P, De Cristofaro R. Radiographic and computed tomographic findings in hydatid disease of bone. Skelet Radiol 1990;19(6): 435–9.

[27] Richter J, Hatz C, Haussinger D. Ultrasound in tropical and parasitic diseases. Lancet 2003;362(9387):900–2

[28] Kalinova K. Imaging (ultrasonography, computed tomography) of patients with hydatid liver disease. Bulgarian Journal of Veterinary Medicine (2007), 10, No 1, 45–51

[29] Filippou D, Tselepis D, Filippou G, Papadopoulos V. Advances in liver echinococcosis: diagnosis and treatment. *Clin Gastroenterol Hepatol* 2007; 5: 152-159

[30] Mortelé KJ, Ros PR. Cystic focal liver lesions in the adult: differential CT and MR imaging features. *Radiographics* 2001; 21: 895-910

[31] Pedrosa I, Saíz A, Arrazola J, Ferreirós J, Pedrosa CS. Hydatid disease: radiologic and pathologic features and complications. *Radiographics* 2000; 20: 795-817

[32] Lim JH. Parasitic diseases in the abdomen: imaging findings. *Abdom Imaging* 2008; 33: 130-132

[33] Magistrelli P, Masetti r, Coppola R, Messia A. Surgical treatment of hydatid disease of liver: a 20 year experience. Arch Surg 1991; 126:518–523.

[34] Zaouche A, Haouet K. Traitement chirurgical des kystes hydatiques du foie. EMC, Techniques chirurgicales, Appareil digestif. Elsevier Masson ; 40-775.

[35] *Balik A. et al.* Surgical Treatment of Hydatid Disease of the Liver Review of 304 Cases. *Arch Surg. 1999;134:166-169.*

[36] Giordano G, Angrisano A, Palazzo P. *et al.* Surgical treatment of hydatid cyst of the liver: pericystectomy or resection. Personal experience. *Int J Surg Sci.* 1999;6: 113-7

[37] M.A. Silva D.F. Mirza S.R. Bramhall A.D. Mayer P. McMaster J.A.C. Buckels. Treatment of Hydatid Disease of the Liver .Evaluation of a UK Experience Dig Surg 2004;21:227–234

[38] Orhan Elbir et al. Surgical Treatment of Intrabiliary Rupture of Hydatid Cysts of Liver: Comparison of Choledochoduodenostomy with T-Tube Drainage. Dig Surg 2001;18:289–293

[39] Perdromo R, Morelli R, Carrquiry L, Chifflet J, Berragalli L. Cholédocostomie transhépaticokystique en cas de kyste hydatique ouvert dans les voies biliaires. Presse Med 1977; 6:747-749.

[40] Saglam A. Laparoscopic treatment of liver hydatid cysts. Surg Lap Endosc 1996; 6:16–21.

[41] Metin Ertem, Tayfun Karahasanoglu, Nihat Yavuz, Sabri Erguney, Laparoscopically Treated Liver Hydatid Cysts Arch Surg. 2002;137:1170-1173

[42] Hesham Maged Hasan , Osama Mahmoud El-Sayed. Laproscopic treatment of liver hydatid cyst. Journal of Medicine and Biomedical Sciences, ISSN: 2078-0273, May, 2010

[43] Skroubis G, Vagianos C, Polydorou A. *et al*. Significance of bile leaks complicating conservative surgery for liver hydatidosis. *World J Surg*.2002;26:704-8
[44] Ersan O, Yusuf B. Endoscopic therapy in the management of hepatobiliary hydatid disease. J Clin Gastrienterol 2002;35:160-174.
[45] Saritas U, Parlak E, Akoglu E, Sahin B. Effectiveness of endoscopic treatment modalities in complicated hepatic hydatid disease after surgical intervention. Endoscopy 2001;33: 858-863.
[46] Palez V, Kugler C, Correa D, Carpio MD. PAIR as percutaneous treatment of hydatid liver cysts. Acta Tropica 2000; 75:197–202.
[47] Yaghan R, Heis H, Bani-Hani K, et al. Is fear of anaphylactic shock discouraging surgeons from more widely adopting percutaneous and laparoscopic techniques in the treatment of liver hydatid cyst? *Am J Surg* 2004; 187:533–537
[48] Ben Amor N, Gargouri M, Gharbi HA, Golvan YJ, Ayachi K, Kchouck H. Trial therapy of inoperable abdominal hydatid cysts by puncture. *Ann Parasitol Hum Comp* 1986; 61:689–692
[49] Giorgio A, Tarantino L, Francica G, et al. Unilocular hydatid liver cysts: treatment with US guided, double percutaneous aspiration and alcohol injection. *Radiology* 1992; 184:705–710
[50] Khuroo MS, Wani NA, Javid G, et al. Percutaneous drainage compared with surgery for hepatic hydatid cysts. *N Engl J Med* 1997; 337:881–887
[51] Kabaalioglu A, Ceken K, Alimoglu E, Apaydin A. Percutaneous imaging-guided treatment of hydatid liver cysts: do long-term results make it a first choice? *Eur J Radiol* 2006; 59:65–73
[52] Antonio Giorgio, Antonella Di Sarno, Giorgio de Stefano, Giulia Liorre Nunzia, Farella Umberto Scognamiglio, Valentina Giorgio. Sonography and Clinical Outcome of Viable Hydatid Liver Cysts Treated With Double Percutaneous Aspiration and Ethanol Injection as First-Line Therapy: Efficacy and Long-Term Follow-Up- *AJR* 2009; 193:186–192
[53] V. Pelaez , C. Kugler, D. Correa, M. Del Carpio, M. Guangiroli, J. Molina, B. Marcos, E. Lopez. PAIR as percutaneous treatment of hydatid liver cysts.Acta Tropica 75 (2000) 197–202
[54] PAIR: Puncture, Aspiration, Injection, Re-Aspiration- An option for the treatment of Cystic Echinococcosis World Health Organization. WHO/CDS/CSR/APH/2001.6
[55] Sakhri J., Ben Ali A. Le kyste hydatique du foie. J. Chir 2004,141(6), 381-9
[56] Ben Amor N, Gargouri M, Gharbi HA, Golvan YJ, Ayachi K, Kchouk KH.. Essai de traitement par ponction des kystes hydatiques abdominaux inopérables. *Ann Parasitol Hum Comp*, 1986; 61: 689-692.
[57] Ben Amor N, Gargouri M, Gharbi HA, Golvan YJ, Ayachi K, Kcouck H. Percutaneous treatment of hydatid cysts under sonographic guidance. *Digestive Diseases and Sciences*, 1994; 39: 1576-1580.
[58] Aktan AO, Yalin R. Preoperative albendazole treatment for liver hydatid disease decreases the viability of the cyst. *Eur J Gastroenterol Hepatol*. 1996;8 877-879.

[59] Blanton RE, Wachira TM, Zeyhle EE, Njoroge EM, Magambo JK, Schantz PM. Oxfendazole treatment for cystic hydatid disease in naturally infected animals. *Antimicrob Agents Chemother*. 1998;42:601-605.

[60] Dziri C, Haouet K, Fingerhut A. Treatment of hydatid cyst of the liver: where is the evidence? *World J Surg* 2004; 28:731–736

Chapter 6

Abdominal Advanced Oncologic Surgery

Enrico Maria Pasqual and Serena Bertozzi

Additional information is available at the end of the chapter

http://dx.doi.org/10.5772/48155

1. Introduction

1.1. The peritoneal cavity, locoregional area

The peritoneal cavity, enclosed by visceral and parietal peritoneum , is the largest potential space in the body. With its own vascularization and lymphatic drainage, is anatomically separated from the general body system and other body compartments.

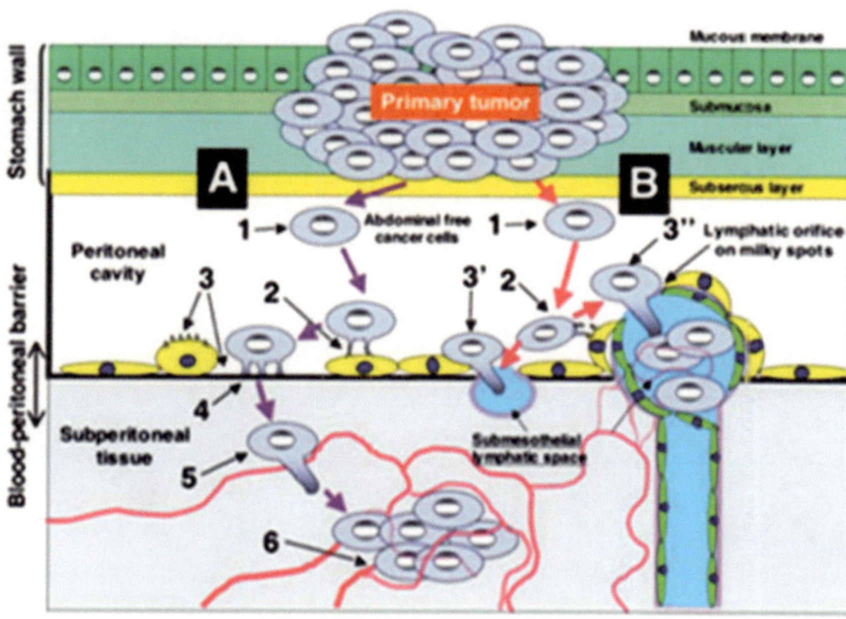

Figure 1. Mechanisms of peritoneal cancer cells seeding.

Any pathological process involving the peritoneal cavity can easily disseminate throughout this space by means of unrestricted movement of fluid and cells. Accordingly malignant intraperitoneal tumour progression, before reaching the circulation system and developing distant metastases (pulmonary, brain and bone metastases) diffuses within and through the peritoneal cavity (Fig. 1). At this step intraperitoneal tumours must be considered in locoregional stage.

Peritoneal neoplasia can originate de novo from the peritoneal tissues (primary tumour) or invade or metastasize into the peritoneum from adjacent or remote organs (metastases).

Rare are the primitive tumours of the peritoneum: they include malignant mesothelioma, peritoneal primary carcinoma and sarcoma.

Malignant peritoneal mesothelioma is a rare but aggressive tumor derived from the peritoneal mesothelium accounting for 2 cases per 1 million population reported each year in USA. Association of malignant peritoneal mesothelioma and asbestos exposure has been reported to be as high as 83%. This locally aggressive disease is difficult to treat or palliate. Commonly, treatment regimens combine aggressive cytoreductive surgery with intraperitoneal chemotherapy. Cytoreductive surgery is the cornerstone of current treatment, while hyperthermic intraoperative intraperitoneal chemotherapy (HIPEC) is a promising strategy in suitable patients (Deraco *et al.*, 2002) (Fig. 2).

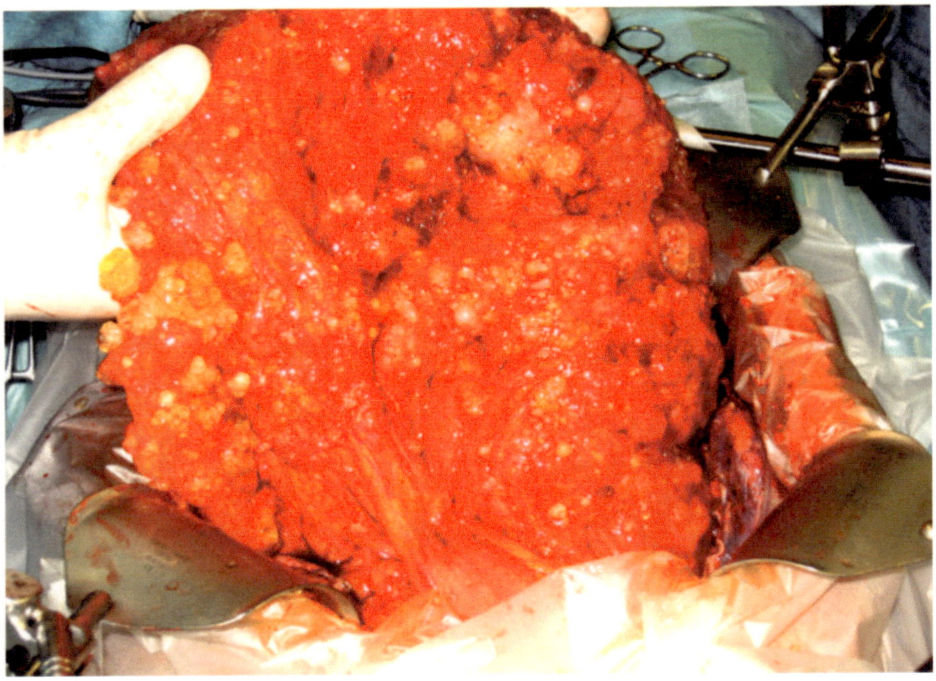

Figure 2. Omental cake.

Primary peritoneal carcinoma is a very rare tumour and (ie, serous surface papillary carcinoma) arises primarily from peritoneal cells. This malignancy predominantly affects postmenopausal women and typically displays multicentric peritoneal and omental involvement. Pathologically and clinically, it resembles papillary serous ovarian carcinoma.

Many primary tumours, arising from organs placed within the peritoneal cavity, disseminate through it, leading patients to death. Peritoneal cavity represents the site of metastases in 50% of colorectal cancer, 50% of gastric cancer and 75% of ovarian advanced cancer. It represents the sole site of intraperitoneal metastasis in 20-25% of colorectal cancer, 30% of gastric cancer and 70% of ovarian cancer (Koppe *et al.*, 2006; Randall and Rubin, 2001; Sadeghi *et al.*, 2000). Intraperitoneal drug administration studies confirmed the existence of a peritoneal-plasma barrier which allows to concentrate the antiblastic drug within the cavity even 100-1000 times compared with that of the same drug infused through systemic circulation. Therefore a high antiblastic tumour tissue concentration and a low systemic toxicity can be achieved (Flessner, 2005). In association with intraperitoneal chemotherapy, hyperthermia has been demonstrated to enhance drug diffusion within the tumour tissue and also to have a direct antitumour activity (Issels, 2008) (Fig. 3)

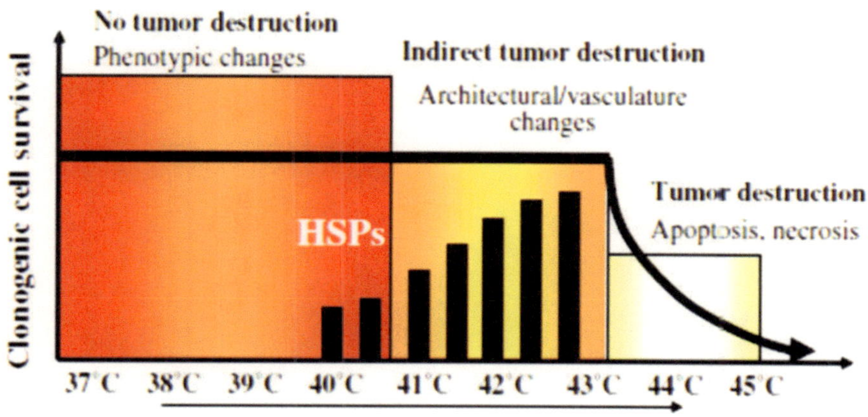

Molecular response	Cell cycle: DNA repair Apoptosis/Necrosis Induction of heat shock proteins/HSP-70 membrane expression
Clinical setting	Thermosensitisation for chemotherapy and/or radiation

Figure 3. Hyperthermia effects on tumour cells.

Therefore cytoreduction and HIPEC procedure have been suggested to treat metastases from colorectal , gastric and gynaecological tumors (Sugarbaker, 1995). Results after treatment are encouraging in particular in cases of colorectal and gynaecological cancer with median 5 years survival respectively of 40% and 45%. Less satisfactory results have been obtained in case of gastric and pancreatic cancer with a minimal percentage of patient still living far from initial diagnosis (Elias *et al.*, 2006; Roviello *et al.*, 2011). The aggressive tumour surgical removal (tumour cytoreduction) coupled with intraperitoneal chemotherapy nowadays represents the cornerstone of advanced abdominal oncologic surgery (Glehen *et al.*, 2006; Glockzin *et al.*, 2009). A large international experience was therefore made through the last decades with the goal of allowing treatment and possibly cure of intraperitoneal tumours in advanced stage (Levine *et al.*, 2007; Roviello *et al.*, 2011).

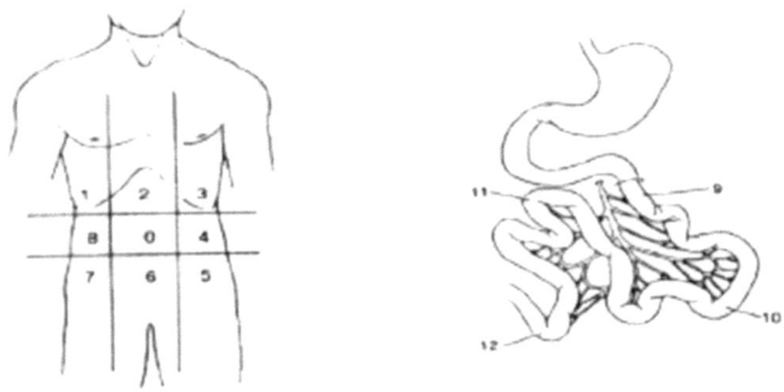

Regions		Lesion Size	Lesion SizeScore (the largest implants scored in each regions)
0	central	________	LS 0 No tumor seen
1	Right upper	________	LS 1 ≤ 0.5 cm
2	Epigastrium	________	LS 2 > 0.5 cm to ≤ 5.0 cm
3	Left upper	________	LS 3 > 5 cm or confluence
4	Left flank	________	
5	Left lower	________	
6	Pelvis	________	
7	Right lower	________	
8	Right flank	________	
9	Upper jejunum	________	
10	Lower jejunum	________	
11	Upper ileum	________	
12	Lower ileum	________	
	PCI	0-39	

Figure 4. Peritoneal cancer index to map carcinosis localization.

2. Cytoreduction and intraperitoneal hyperthermic chemotherapy (HIPEC)

Advanced metastatic tumour can therefore be treated with surgery and hyperthermic chemotherapy contemporarily, during the same surgical operating work up. The first step is to carry out an aggressive cytoreduction in order to remove the whole macroscopic intracavitary tumour tissue and then to complete the procedure with HIPEC, to kill residual neoplastic cells floating within the peritoneal cavity or adherent to intraperitoneal tissue.

2.1. Cytoreduction

The surgical procedure of cytoreduction is now well standardized . Sugarbaker's classification is still the reference for abdominal oncologic surgery and goes under the definition of peritonectomy. The surgical procedure was classified according to specific different areas of the abdominal cavity and it has been tailored by Milan 's panel workshop, defining (Fig. 4):

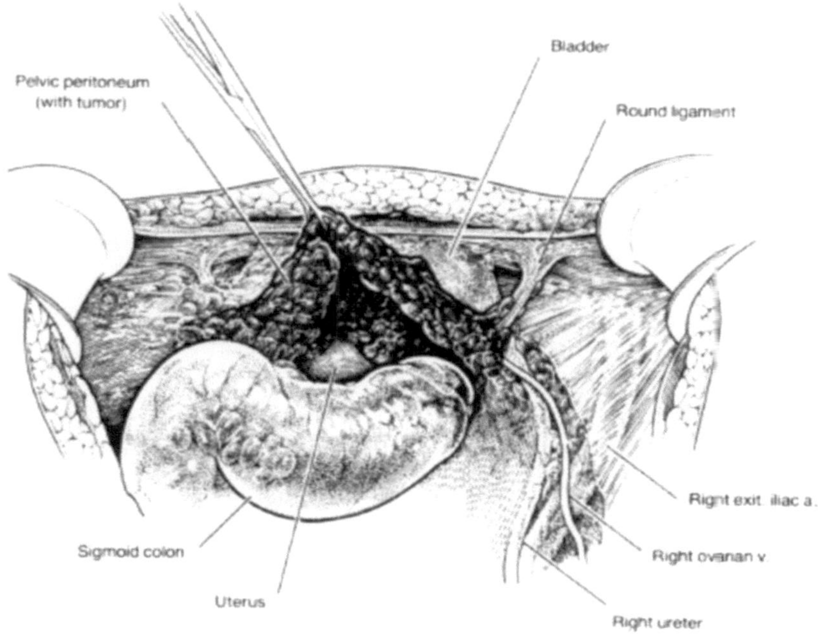

Figure 5. Surgical cytoreduction.

1. Upper RightPeritonectomy: right diaphragmatic peritonectomy with Glisson's capsule dissection; lesser omentectomy, stripping of the omental bursa and cholecystectomy plus gastric antrectomy or total gastrectomy.
2. Upper Left Peritonectomy: left diaphragmatic and parietal peritonectomy with splenectomy and greater omentectomy.
3. Pelvic Peritonectomy: pelvic parietal peritonectomy, sigmoidectomy, hysterectomy and salpingo-ovariectomy.
4. Right Parietal Peritonectomy, right/total colectomy; left parietal peritonectomy.
5. Mesenteric implants on visceral surfaces could be removed surgically or by electrosurgical local dissection. Performing cytoreduction for peritoneal tumour dissemination, not all the procedures are necessary and made, usually necessitating one – three of the different peritonectomy procedures (Fig. 4 and 5).

2.2. Intraperitoneal hyperthermic chemotherapy

After having made complete surgical cytoreduction with an absent or minimal residual disease (less than 2.5 mm tumour diameter) some catheters are inserted into the abdominal cavity and a perfusion of 2 liters of a saline solution with a determined quantity of antiblastic drug (Mytomycin, Oxaliplatin for digestive cancer and Cisplatin, Taxol for ovarian cancer) is made . The peritoneal perfusion may lasts 30-90 minutes and it can be performed in condition of closed abdomen or open abdomen (Coliseum technique) or a compromise between the two, with an abdominal- wall small entrance suitable for the handling by the operator. (Fig. 6).

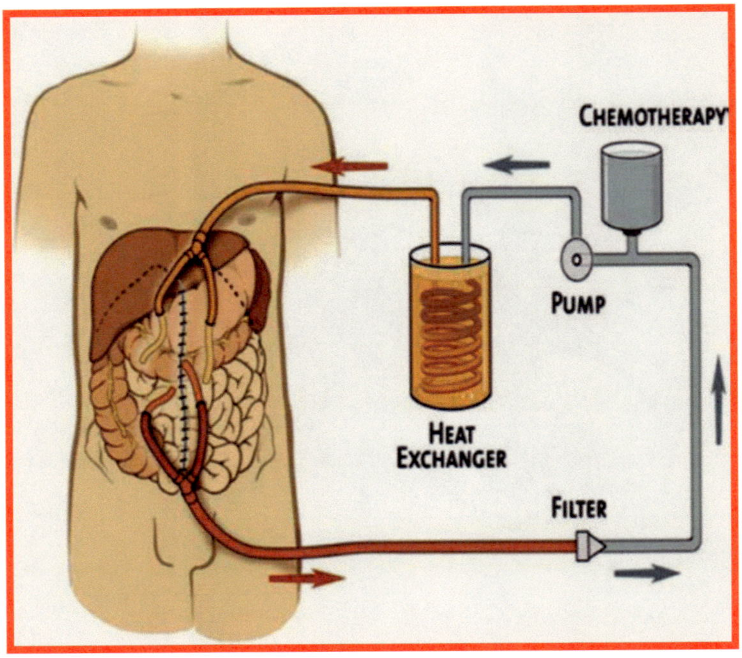

Figure 6. Hyperthermic intraperitoneal chemotherapy

Hyperthermic perfusion can be obtained by heating the perfusion medium with a heat exchanger connected to the perfusion pump. The peritoneal cavity temperature considered optimal in terms of antitumor activity and antiblastic tumour tissue diffusion is 41,5-42,5 °C (Sugarbaker and Chang, 1999; Sugarbaker, 1996; Van der Speeten *et al.*, 2009). It is of absolute importance to control the temperature of organs and bowels during the procedure. Excessive temperature of intraperitoneal tissue, more than 43 °C, is strongly correlated with lesions of the bowel wall and perforation, and also with necrosis of nerves, bladder or vases. To prevent excessive intraperitoneal temperature multiple temperature probes are placed within the peritoneal cavity to monitorate the temperature. At the end of the procedure the perfused medium is usually removed from the peritoneal cavity.

3. Advanced oncological surgery in colorectal cancer

Every year about 400.000 new cases of colorectal cancer (CRC) are diagnosed in Europe and 210.000 are believed to die of disease (Boyle and Ferlay, 2005). Peritoneal carcinosis (PC) has an incidence about 13% of CRC, in 58% of cases is synchronus with primary disease and in most cases is not diffused to the entire abdominal cavity but limited to an area (Jayne *et al.*, 2002). Peritoneal cavity recurrence is the only site of relapse in about 25% of cases (Chu *et al.*, 1989). The principal mechanism of peritoneal cancer diffusion through the abdominal cavity is the esfoliation of cancer cells following bowel-serosa tumour infiltration. Also lymphatic channel infiltration by the tumour followed by breaking of the lymphatic channel wall and subsequently loss of neoplastic cells within the abdominal cavity is a mechanism of PC formation. Furthermore at the time of surgical work up tumour manipulation and blood loss are also intracavitary mechanism of PC formation. Facing PC, both synchronous or metachronous, the usual treatment is systemic chemotherapy but median survival is usually not longer than 6 months even after the advent of new drugs and treatment scheme (Sadeghi *et al.*, 2000). More recently Dominique Elias has published an experience with patients with PC and absence of extra-abdominal disease by using modern scheme of chemotherapy FOLFOX (5-FU, AF and oxaliplatin) and FOLFIRI (5-FU, AF and irinotecan) obtaining a median survival of 23,9 months and a 2 and 5 years survival of 65% and 13% respectively (Elias *et al.*, 2009). The advent of CRS with HIPEC have ameliorated the prognosis in these patients (Elias *et al.*, 2006; Verwaal *et al.*, 2005; Yan and Morris, 2008).

During the last decade a randomized study , two multicentric comparative studies and a numbers of observational studies have tested the CRS and HIPEC activity against PC from CRC with encouraging results: mortality and postoperative morbidity of 0-8% and 39-72% respectively and 5 years survival of 40-51% (Verwaal *et al.*, 2003, 2005; Elias *et al.*, 2009, 2006; Franko *et al.*, 2010). Main indications for application of the procedure are the presence of PC both synchronous or metachronous , therefore defining it a therapeutic procedure. But recent experiences also suggest the possible use of HIPEC in adjuvant setting after radical surgery work up. Not all patients with CRC could benefits from this approach. A number of risk factors for PC development have been demonstrated: minimal PC which was macroscopically visible, completely resected or ovarian metastasis (also resected), synchronous with the primary tumour or a perforated primary tumor inside the peritoneal cavity, primary CRC presenting with occlusion or haemorrhagia. Patients bearing these risk factors and treated with cytoreduction and HIPEC at the end of cytoreduction (no residual tumour disease was present - R0 resection) showed, in preliminary experiences, impressive results with a 5 years survival percentage reaching 90% and a 5 years disease free survival of more than 40% (Elias *et al.*, 2009). This preliminary experience supports a large number of multi-istitutional ongoing worldwide studies to confirm the role of cytoreduction and hyperthermic intraperitoneal chemoperfusion in adjuvant setting at the same time of primary surgery or after a planned second look exploration. This new therapeutic approach even if after a long maturation phase lasting more than a decade, now seems to be accepted as a new frontier to treat advanced CRC and world wide surgical units have been created to coordinate and carry on the associated medical activity.

4. Advanced oncological surgery in gastric cancer

PC from gastric cancer arises following tumours invasion of the gastric serosa as depicted in Fig. 7. Also histological type can be crucial in PC gastric developing. Gastric tumours of the diffused type seems to represent a risk factor for PC and it has been demonstrated to relapse in about 50% of cases even after curative surgical resection (Marrelli *et al.*, 2002). It has been shown that the serosal tumor invasion is correlated to the detection rate of intraperitoneal free cancer cells. The treatment of peritoneal carcinomatosis from gastric cancer by peritonectomy and HIPEC has demonstrated not so good long-term results when compared with the treatment of PC from other causes (Stewart *et al.*, 2005). Anyway conventional treatment using palliative systemic chemotherapy showed a very dismal prognosis

(Hanazaki *et al.*, 1999). Long survival after peritonectomy and HIPEC for carcinomatosis arising from gastric cancer are possible if the extension of the carcinosis is low and the cytoreduction is complete. 3-year survival of 41% and 5-year survival rates of 11% was reported (Sayag-Beaujard *et al.*, 1999; Yonemura *et al.*, 2001, 1996). CRS and HIPEC of the PC seems to allow longer survival even if hyperthermic intraperitoneal chemoperfusion role is still under evaluation.

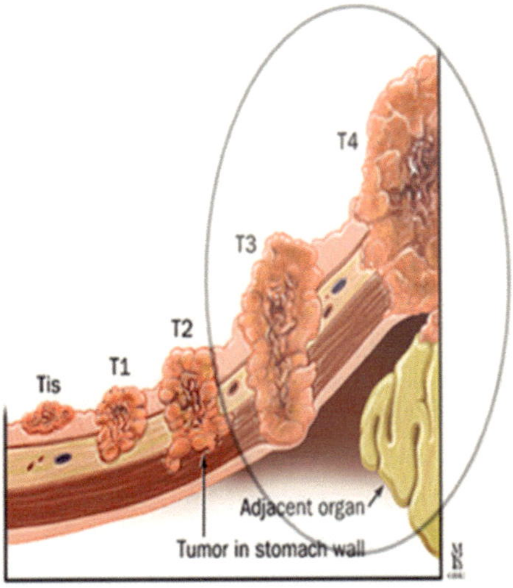

Figure 7. Invasion of the gastric serosa.

Recent experiences with HIPEC have shown quite encouraging results in case of prevention of peritoneal recurrence after radical surgery for primary carcinoma, the adjuvant role. When curative gastrectomy is performed, in fact, peritoneal recurrence develops in nearly 50% of patients , therefore prevention of PC developing represent a fundamental goal in this setting (Yonemura *et al.*, 2001, 1996; Fujimoto *et al.*, 1999; Shen *et al.*, 2009). Worldwide experiences are ongoing to ascertain the role of HIPEC in adjuvant setting and definitive results will be available in a short time.

5. Advanced oncological surgery in ovarian cancer

Epithelial ovarian cancers account for 80% to 90% of all ovarian malignancies and are the main cause of death for all gynaecological tumors (Yancik, 1993). Despite being diagnosed frequently at an advanced stage, dissemination is often confined to the peritoneal cavity (Randall and Rubin, 2001). It presents with vague gastrointestinal and constitutional symptoms of abdominal bloating, distension, weight loss, and fatigue (Goff *et al.*, 2000). Late presentation results in the majority of patients being diagnosed with advanced disease (Stage III/IV). The 5-year survival rate of patients with advanced ovarian cancer is <25% (Ozols, 2005). In the final stages of this disease, patients suffer from severe anorexia, dyspnea and pain from malignant bowel obstruction, ascites, and pleural effusion as a result of the extensive burden of tumor.

Epithelial ovarian tumor arises from the serosal lining of the ovary. This covering of the ovary communicates with the serosal lining of the abdominopelvic cavity, and is known as the peritoneum. Tumor growth results in the exfoliation of malignant cells into the peritoneal fluid. They circulate freely and typically implant in the pelvis and subdiaphramatic recesses owing to gravity and the incumbent position Intraoperatively, it is characterized by the extensive presence of macroscopic whitish tumor nodules of variable sizes and consistency that may coalesce to form plaques or masses within the abdominopelvic cavity.

Tumor dissemination from the primary tumour may also occur through the lymphatic channel disrupted by the tumour and the direction of neoplastic cell diffusion is all through the abdominal cavity.

CRS using limited peritonectomy procedures to resect peritoneal implants and HIPEC aims to allow both macroscopic cytoreduction through surgery and cytotoxic cytoreduction through loco-regional administration of heated chemotherapy. Cytoreduction and HIPEC has been tested in different routes; front line when treating the primary cancer, as interval surgery after neoadjuvat chemotherapy in case of unresectable cancer, as treatment of ovarian cancer relapses and even in case of salvage therapy (Look *et al.*, 2004).

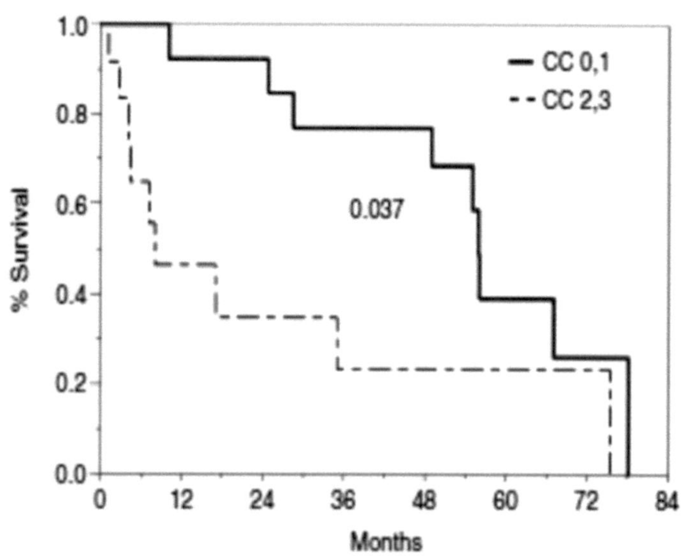

Figure 8. Ovarian cancer survival in compete and non complete cytoreduction.

The largest experience to date was reported by Bereder who reported a median overall survival of 46 months in patients with first relapsed ovarian cancer of which a proportion are chemoresistant. In their institutions, the mortality rate was under 1% and the morbidity rates were about 10%.The treatment related complications is considered acceptable and further large volume peritonectomy units have low morality rates that range from 0 to 2% (Raspagliesi *et al.*, 2006; Bereder *et al.*, 2009; Look *et al.*, 2004). Nowadays there is large agreement on the role of extreme cytoreduction of peritoneal carcinosis in case of ovarian cancer. Two groups of patients are then obtained: those with residual disease no more than 2.5 mm in diameter corresponding to the completeness cytoreduction rate CC0-1 and those with residual disease more than 2.5 mm CC2-3. The first group with a complete tumour eradication shows a significative better survival (Fig. 8).

Promising results have been published during this decade improving survival and disease free survival. This particular indication for this complex procedure represents a very promising but also conflicting tool because of the high drug Platinum sensitivity of ovarian cancer which makes medical oncologist to be confident with systemic chemotherapy results. Unfortunately despite a great number of patients optimally treated in this way a significant fraction of them relapse (50-70%) and in this case it is reasonable to think that extreme cytoreduction and HIPEC can be helpful.

6. Advanced oncological surgery in malignant peritoneal mesothelioma

Diffuse malignant peritoneal mesothelioma (DMPM) is a relatively uncommon peritoneal malignancy, representing 20-30% of 2.200-2.500 new cases diagnosed every year in USA, but its incidence has been rising worldwide since 1970s and is not expected to peak for another 5 to 20 years. The reason lays in its recognized association with asbestos exposure, which has been extensively used in the past as building material (Battifora, 1995; Robinson and Lake, 2005). Along with the occupational exposure, DMPM has been reported following radiation therapy, mica exposure, recurrent peritonitis and thorium dioxide administration (Maurer and Egloff, 1975; Antman *et al.*, 1983; Chahinian *et al.*, 1982; Riddell *et al.*, 1981).

It is characterized macroscopically by thousands of whitish tumor nodules of variable size and consistency that may coalesce to form plaques or masses that may layer out to uniformly cover the entire peritoneal surface. Traditionally, DMPM was considered a preterminal condition, as the majority of patients died from intestinal obstruction or terminal starvation within the first year from the diagnosis (Yan *et al.*, 2007). Despite its generally local spread without lymphoadenopathy or distant organ metastases, its poor prognosis may be explained by late diagnosis, due to the aspecificity of presenting symptoms (abdominal pain, girth, ascitis,...) and the inadequateness of most imaging tools in detecting small nodules on the whole peritoneal surface. Furthermore, no uniform treatment was initially suggested for this kind of malignancy, systemic chemotherapy and abdominal radiation therapy showed scarce results and were used only in selected patients, and surgery had only a palliative role to resolve intestinal obstruction in urgency without any significant effect on patients prognosis (Chailleux *et al.*, 1988; Antman *et al.*, 1983; Eltabbakh *et al.*, 1999; Markman and Kelsen, 1992; Neumann *et al.*, 1999; Sridhar *et al.*, 1992; Yates *et al.*, 1997). Recently, diagnostic and therapeutic aspects of the disease have been re-evaluated as encouraging reports from several centers worldwide on a combined locoregional treatment approach that uses cytoreductive surgery (CRS) and hyperthermic intraperitoneal chemotherapy (HIPEC) have emerged. This new treatment strategy has shown favorable prognosis and has achieved in selected patients a median survival of up to

60 months and a 5-year survival of 50% using different antiblastic sequence (Deraco *et al.*, 2006; Nonaka *et al.*, 2005; Park *et al.*, 1999; Sugarbaker *et al.*, 2003; Yan *et al.*, 2007).

Given its tendency to remain confined to the peritoneal surface, the prognosis of DMPM has been significantly improved by the combined treatment with CRS and HIPEC. In particular, while CRS reduces the tumoral mass (an optimal cytoreduction aims to residual disease smaller than 2,5mm), HIPEC maximizes loco-regional chemotherapy cytotoxicity while limiting the systemic side effects (Vlasveld *et al.*, 1991; Markman, 1990; Markman and Kelsen, 1992). In this perspective, some encouraging experiences in numerous centers demonstrated a median survival of 40 to 90 months and a 5-ys-OS of 30 to 60% (Yan *et al.*, 2007; Brigand *et al.*, 2006; Deraco *et al.*, 2006; Feldman *et al.*, 2003; Loggie *et al.*, 2001; Nonaka *et al.*, 2005; Park *et al.*, 1999; Sugarbaker *et al.*, 2003). All peritonetomy center agree that complete cytoreduction is the prognostic principal factor for clinical success and that complete cytoreduction is correlated to the initial extent of intrabdominal disease and to the ability of the surgical team. Despite the data available, the role of HIPEC in this setting represents one of the strongest indications, particularly in view of considerable survival improvement over the best systemic therapy to date offered (Munkholm-Larsen *et al.*, 2009; Shen *et al.*, 2009).

7. Advanced oncological surgery in pseudomyxoma peritonei

Appendiceal tumors are uncommon neoplasms accounting for about 1% of all colorectal malignancies.

The majority of appendix cancers are carcinoid tumors; the second most common are epithelial neoplasms. The latter frequently present with mucinous ascites and mucinous tumor implants throughout the abdominal cavity. Such rare condition, with an incidence of approximately 1/1,000,000/year, is known as pseudomyxoma peritonei (PMP). Mucinous adenocarcinoma originating from large bowel, ovary, or other intra-abdominal sites may mimic PMP (Baratti *et al.*, 2008). According to Ronnett, PMP was histologically classified into disseminated peritoneal adenomucinosis (DPAM), peritoneal mucinous carcinomatosis (PMCA), and intermediate or discordant feature group (ID). Appendiceal tumors were classified into low-grade appendiceal mucinous neoplasm (LAMN) and mucinous adenocarcinoma (MACA) (Misdraji). Pseudomyxoma peritonei (PMP) represents a rare peritoneal malignancy with a controversial bordeline behavior. Although a possible ovarian origin was initially suggested in the female sex, the over-expression of determined molecular markers has finally demonstrated a more probable PMP origin from a perforated appendiceal epithelial tumor. Undoubtedly, a small proportion of cases originate anyway from other organs, which ovarian primary is likely to be the more commonest of, followed by colon and rectum, stomach, gallbladder and biliary ducts, small bowel, urinary bladder, lung, breast, falloppian tube and pancreas (Smeenk *et al.*, 2006, 2007; de Bree *et al.*, 2000).

PMP is clinically characterized by diffuse intra-abdominal gelatinous collections with mucinous implants on peritoneal surfaces. Its pathognomonic accumulation at specific abdominal and pelvic sites is due to the so-called phenomenon of "redistribution" within the peritoneal cavity, which is determined by physical factors, such as the movement and absorption of peritoneal fluid and gravity (Sugarbaker, 1994). Despite its usually indolent behavior, its natural history is characterized by a slow progression to terminal starvation through intestinal obstruction by mucinous ascitis. Recent pathological (Ronnett *et al.*, 1995) molecular genetic (Szych *et al.*, 1999) and immunohistochemical studies (Carr *et al.*, 2002) have provided substantial evidence that most cases of PMP originate from ruptured low grade appendiceal tumors and that mucin-producing epithelial cells accumulate into the abdominal cavity as a result of a distribution process.Therefore, surgical management consisted in repeated interval debulking for symptomatic relief (Sugarbaker, 1996). Based on recent prospective trials, CRS and HIPEC has been proposed as the standard of care for PMP. Results are encouraging with a 5-ys-OS ranging from 62.5 to 100% for low grade PMP and from 0 to 65% for high grade disease . This differentiation is crucial for the evolution of disease; low grade tumours are slow growing and indolent differently from those high grade, fast growing and aggressive (Sugarbaker and Chang, 1999; Witkamp *et al.*, 2001; Güner *et al.*, 2005; Moran *et al.*, 2008; Moran and Cecil, 2003; Murphy *et al.*, 2007; Baratti *et al.*, 2008; Elias *et al.*, 2008; Loungnarath *et al.*, 2005; Smeenk *et al.*, 2007; Stewart *et al.*, 2005; Yan *et al.*, 2006). The goal of the surgical cytoreduction is to remove all the visible tumor by the following procedures: right subdiaphragmatic and parietal peritonectomy, left subdiaphragmatic and parietal peritonectomy,greater omentectomy with splenectomy, lesser omentectomy and stripping of the omental bursa, andpelvic peritonectomy with salpingo-oophorectomy in women. Depending on disease extent, implants on visceral serosa were removed by electrosurgical local dissection or multivisceral resections including Glisson's capsule dissection, cholecystectomy, partial or total gastrectomy, sigmoid, right or total colectomy. According to several phase I and II prospective trials, 5-year survivals have ranged between 66% and 97% (Stewart *et al.*, 2005). It must be taken in mind that, because of the limited data on prognostic factors for this procedure in the setting of appendiceal primary tumors, further well designed, prospective, multi-institutional study are required (Bevan *et al.*, 2010; Roviello *et al.*, 2011).

8. Conclusion

CRS and HIPEC is a complex therapeutic systems which require highly specialized human resources, complex technological facilities, very much depending from expertize of the team involved. Literature refers to a learning curve of more than 100 procedures underscoring the crucial importance of treatment center experience. A continuous comparison must be done with new systemic and locoregional treatment possibility in order to verify new advantages in term of patient survival. This is the reason why a biannual international meeting is planned for comparing results, verify indications and planning of further studies regard to indications, duration and temperature of the perfusion, open or closed perfusion models or type and dosage of chemotherapeutic agents.

The future of treatment of peritoneal carcinosis appears correlated to the strong cooperation with medical oncologists to select patients and focusing on the timing of treatment which in our experience is crucial. The development of new scheme treatment must be approached as in treating ovarian peritoneal carcinosis with front line, interval, or salvage procedures.

Therefore creating regional centers dedicated to peritoneal carcinosis treatment that investigate not only response and survival, but also standardization of technique and methods to do CRS and deliver HIPEC remains crucial.

Author details

Enrico Maria Pasqual and Serena Bertozzi
University of Udine, Italy

9. References

Antman K, Shemin R, Ryan L, Klegar K, Osteen R, Herman T, Lederman G, Corson J. Malignant mesothelioma: prognostic variables in a registry of 180 patients, the Dana-Farber Cancer Institute and Brigham and Women's Hospital experience over two decades, 1965-1985. J Clin Oncol 1988; 6:147-153;

Antman KH, Corson JM, Li FP, Greenberger J, Sytkowski A, Henson DE, Weinstein L. Malignant mesothelioma following radiation exposure. *J Clin Oncol* 1983;1:695–700.

Baratti D, Kusamura S, Nonaka D, Langer M, Andreola S, Favaro M, Gavazzi C, Laterza B, Deraco M. Pseudomyxoma peritonei: clinical pathological and biological prognostic factors in patients treated with cytoreductive surgery and hyperthermic intraperitoneal chemotherapy (HIPEC). *Ann Surg Oncol* 2008;15:526–534.

Battifora H. Tumors of the serosal membranes. Armed Forces Institute of Pathology under the auspices of Universities Associated for Research and Education in Pathology, Washington, D.C, 1995.

Bereder J, Glehen O, Habre J, Desantis M, Cotte E, Mounier N, Ray-Cocquard I, Karimdjee B, Bakrin N, Bernard J, *et al.* Cytoreductive surgery combined with perioperative intraperitoneal chemotherapy for the management of peritoneal carcinomatosis from ovarian cancer: a multiinstitutional study of 246 patients. In *J Clin Oncol* (Meeting Abstracts), vol. 27. 2009; 5542.

Bevan KE, Mohamed F, Moran BJ. Pseudomyxoma peritonei. *World J Gastrointest Oncol* 2010;2:44–50.

Boyle P, Ferlay J. Cancer incidence and mortality in europe, 2004. *Ann Oncol* 2005;16:481–488.

Brigand C, Monneuse O, Mohamed F, Sayag-Beaujard AC, Isaac S, Gilly FN, Glehen O. Peritoneal mesothelioma treated by cytoreductive surgery and intraperitoneal hyperthermic chemotherapy: results of a prospective study. *Ann Surg Oncol* 2006;13:405–412.

Carr NJ, Emory TS, Sobin LH. Epithelial neoplasms of the appendix and colorectum: an analysis of cell proliferation, apoptosis, and expression of p53, cd44, bcl-2. *Arch Pathol Lab Med* 2002;126:837–841.

Chahinian AP, Pajak TF, Holland JF, Norton L, Ambinder RM, Mandel EM. Diffuse malignant mesothelioma. prospective evaluation of 69 patients. *Ann Intern Med* 1982;96:746–755.

Chailleux E, Dabouis G, Pioche D, de Lajartre M, de Lajartre AY, Rembeaux A, Germaud P. Prognostic factors in diffuse malignant pleural mesothelioma. a study of 167 patients. *Chest* 1988;93:159–162.

Chu DZ, Lang NP, Thompson C, Osteen PK, Westbrook KC. Peritoneal carcinomatosis in nongynecologic malignancy. a prospective study of prognostic factors. *Cancer* 1989;63:364–367.

De Bree E, Witkamp AJ, Zoetmulder FA. Peroperative hyperthermic intraperitoneal chemotherapy (HIPEC) for advanced gastric cancer. *Eur J Surg Oncol* 2000;26:630–632.

Deraco M, Gronchi A, Mazzaferro V, Inglese MG, Pennacchioli E, Kusamura S, Rizzi M, Anselmi RA Jr, Vaglini M. Feasibility of peritonectomy associated with intraperitoneal hyperthermic perfusion in patients with pseudomyxoma peritonei. *Tumori* 2002;88:370–375.

Deraco M, Nonaka D, Baratti D, Casali P, Rosai J, Younan R, Salvatore A, Cabras Ad AD, Kusamura S. Prognostic analysis of clinicopathologic factors in 49 patients with diffuse malignant peritoneal mesothelioma treated with cytoreductive surgery and intraperitoneal hyperthermic perfusion. *Ann Surg Oncol* 2006;13:229–237.

Elias D, Honoré C, Ciuchendéa R, Billard V, Raynard B, Lo Dico R, Dromain C, Duvillard P, Goéré D. Peritoneal pseudomyxoma: results of a systematic policy of complete cytoreductive surgery and hyperthermic intraperitoneal chemotherapy. *Br J Surg* 2008;95:1164–1171.

Elias D, Lefevre JH, Chevalier J, Brouquet A, Marchal F, Classe JM, Ferron G, Guilloit JM, Meeus P, Goéré D, Bonastre J. Complete cytoreductive surgery plus intraperitoneal chemohyperthermia with oxaliplatin for peritoneal carcinomatosis of colorectal origin. *J Clin Oncol* 2009;27:681–685.

Elias D, Raynard B, Farkhondeh F, Goéré D, Rouquie D, Ciuchendea R, Pocard M, Ducreux M. Peritoneal carcinomatosis of colorectal origin. *Gastroenterol Clin Biol* 2006;30:1200–1204.

Eltabbakh GH, Piver MS, Hempling RE, Recio FO, Intengen ME. Clinical picture, response to therapy, and survival of women with diffuse malignant peritoneal mesothelioma. *J Surg Oncol* 1999;70:6–12.

Feldman AL, Libutti SK, Pingpank JF, Bartlett DL, Beresnev TH, Mavroukakis SM, Steinberg SM, Liewehr DJ, Kleiner DE, Alexander HR. Analysis of factors associated with outcome in patients with malignant peritoneal mesothelioma undergoing surgical debulking and intraperitoneal chemotherapy. *J Clin Oncol* 2003;21:4560–4567.

Flessner MF. The transport barrier in intraperitoneal therapy. *Am J Physiol Renal Physiol* 2005;288:F433–F442.

Franko J, Ibrahim Z, Gusani NJ, Holtzman MP, Bartlett DL, Zeh HJ 3rd. Cytoreductive surgery and hyperthermic intraperitoneal chemoperfusion versus systemic chemotherapy alone for colorectal peritoneal carcinomatosis. *Cancer* 2010;116:3756–3762.

Fujimoto S, Takahashi M, Mutou T, Kobayashi K, Toyosawa T. Successful intraperitoneal hyperthermic chemoperfusion for the prevention of postoperative peritoneal recurrence in patients with advanced gastric carcinoma. *Cancer* 1999;85:529–534.

Glehen O, Cotte E, Lifante JC, Arvieux C, Moles N, Brigand C, Beaujard AC, François Y, Gilly FN. Peritoneal carcinomatosis in digestive cancers: cytoreductive surgery combined with intraperitoneal chemohyperthermia. The experience in centre hospitalier et universitaire lyon sud (chls). *Acta Chir Belg* 2006;106:285–290.

Glockzin G, Ghali N, Lang SA, Schlitt HJ, Piso P. Results of cytoreductive surgery and hyperthermic intraperitoneal chemotherapy for peritoneal carcinomatosis from colorectal cancer. *J Surg Oncol* 2009;100:306–310.

Goff BA, Mandel L, Muntz HG, Melancon CH. Ovarian carcinoma diagnosis. *Cancer* 2000;89:2068–2075.

Güner Z, Schmidt U, Dahlke MH, Schlitt HJ, Klempnauer J, Piso P. Cytoreductive surgery and intraperitoneal chemotherapy for pseudomyxoma peritonei. *Int J Colorectal Dis* 2005;20:155–160.

Hanazaki K, Mochizuki Y, Machida T, Yokoyama S, Sodeyama H, Sode Y, Wakabayashi M, Kawamura N, Miyazaki T. Post-operative chemotherapy in non-curative gastrectomy for advanced gastric cancer. *Hepatogastroenterology* 1999;46:1238–1243.

Issels RD. Hyperthermia adds to chemotherapy. *Eur J Cancer* 2008;44:2546–2554.

Jayne DG, Fook S, Loi C, Seow-Choen F. Peritoneal carcinomatosis from colorectal cancer. *Br J Surg* 2002;89:1545–1550.

Koppe MJ, Boerman OC, Oyen WJG, Bleichrodt RP. Peritoneal carcinomatosis of colorectal origin: incidence and current treatment strategies. *Ann Surg* 2006;243:212–222.

Levine EA, Stewart JH 4th, Russell GB, Geisinger KR, Loggie BL, Shen P. Cytoreductive surgery and intraperitoneal hyperthermic chemotherapy for peritoneal surface malignancy: experience with 501 procedures. *J Am Coll Surg* 2007;204:943–53; discussion 953–5.

Loggie BW, Fleming RA, McQuellon RP, Russell GB, Geisinger KR, Levine EA. Prospective trial for the treatment of malignant peritoneal mesothelioma. *Am Surg* 2001;67:999–1003.

Look M, Chang D, Sugarbaker PH. Long-term results of cytoreductive surgery for advanced and recurrent epithelial ovarian cancers and papillary serous carcinoma of the peritoneum. *Int J Gynecol Cancer* 2004;14:35–41.

Loungnarath R, Causeret S, Bossard N, Faheez M, Sayag-Beaujard AC, Brigand C, Gilly F, Glehen O. Cytoreductive surgery with intraperitoneal chemohyperthermia for the treatment of pseudomyxoma peritonei: a prospective study. *Dis Colon Rectum* 2005;48:1372–1379.

Markman M. Intraperitoneal belly bath chemotherapy. Percept Press, Chicago, 2nd ed., 1990.

Markman M, Kelsen D. Efficacy of cisplatin-based intraperitoneal chemotherapy as treatment of malignant peritoneal mesothelioma. *J Cancer Res Clin Oncol* 1992;118:547–550.

Marrelli D, Roviello F, de Manzoni G, Morgagni P, Di Leo A, Saragoni L, De Stefano A, Folli S, Cordiano C, Pinto E, IRGfGC. Different patterns of recurrence in gastric cancer depending on lauren's histological type: longitudinal study. *World J Surg* 2002;26:1160–1165.

Maurer R, Egloff B. Malignant peritoneal mesothelioma after cholangiography with thorotrast. *Cancer* 1975;36:1381–1385.

Moran B, Baratti D, Yan TD, Kusamura S, Deraco M. Consensus statement on the loco-regional treatment of appendiceal mucinous neoplasms with peritoneal dissemination (pseudomyxoma peritonei). *J Surg Oncol* 2008;98:277–282.

Moran BJ, Cecil TD. The etiology, clinical presentation, and management of pseudomyxoma peritonei. *Surg Oncol Clin N Am* 2003;12:585–603.

Munkholm-Larsen S, Cao CQ, Yan TD. Malignant peritoneal mesothelioma. *World J Gastrointest Surg* 2009;1:38–48.

Murphy EM, Sexton R, Moran BJ. Early results of surgery in 123 patients with pseudomyxoma peritonei from a perforated appendiceal neoplasm. *Dis Colon Rectum* 2007;50:37–42.

Neumann V, Müller KM, Fischer M. Peritoneal mesothelioma–incidence and etiology. *Pathologe* 1999;20:169–176.

Nonaka D, Kusamura S, Baratti D, Casali P, Cabras AD, Younan R, Rosai J, Deraco M. Diffuse malignant mesothelioma of the peritoneum: a clinicopathological study of 35 patients treated locoregionally at a single institution. *Cancer* 2005;104:2181–2188.

Ozols RF. Treatment goals in ovarian cancer. *Int J Gynecol Cancer* 2005;15 Suppl 1:3–11.

Park BJ, Alexander HR, Libutti SK, Wu P, Royalty D, Kranda KC, Bartlett DL. Treatment of primary peritoneal mesothelioma by continuous hyperthermic peritoneal perfusion (chpp). *Ann Surg Oncol* 1999;6:582–590.

Randall TC, Rubin SC. Cytoreductive surgery for ovarian cancer. *Surg Clin North Am* 2001;81:871–883.

Raspagliesi F, Kusamura S, Campos Torres JC, de Souza GA, Ditto A, Zanaboni F, Younan R, Baratti D, Mariani L, Laterza B, Deraco M. Cytoreduction combined with intraperitoneal hyperthermic perfusion chemotherapy in advanced/recurrent ovarian cancer patients: The experience of national cancer institute of milan. *Eur J Surg Oncol* 2006;32:671–675.

Riddell RH, Goodman MJ, Moossa AR. Peritoneal malignant mesothelioma in a patient with recurrent peritonitis. *Cancer* 1981;48:134–139.

Robinson BWS, Lake RA. Advances in malignant mesothelioma. *N Engl J Med* 2005;353:1591–1603.

Ronnett BM, Zahn CM, Kurman RJ, Kass ME, Sugarbaker PH, Shmookler BM. Disseminated peritoneal adenomucinosis and peritoneal mucinous carcinomatosis. a clinicopathologic analysis of 109 cases with emphasis on distinguishing pathologic features, site of origin, prognosis, and relationship to "pseudomyxoma peritonei". *Am J Surg Pathol* 1995;19:1390–1408.

Roviello F, Caruso S, Marrelli D, Pedrazzani C, Neri A, De Stefano A, Pinto E. Treatment of peritoneal carcinomatosis with cytoreductive surgery and hyperthermic intraperitoneal chemotherapy: state of the art and future developments. *Surg Oncol* 2011;20:e38–e54.

Sadeghi B, Arvieux C, Glehen O, Beaujard AC, Rivoire M, Baulieux J, Fontaumard E, Brachet A, Caillot JL, Faure JL, Porcheron J, Peix JL, François Y, Vignal J, Gilly FN.

Peritoneal carcinomatosis from non-gynecologic malignancies: results of the evocape 1 multicentric prospective study. *Cancer* 2000;88:358–363.

Sayag-Beaujard AC, Francois Y, Glehen O, Sadeghi-Looyeh B, Bienvenu J, Panteix G, Garbit F, Grandclément E, Vignal J, Gilly FN. Intraperitoneal chemo-hyperthermia with Mitomycin C for gastric cancer patients with peritoneal carcinomatosis. *Anticancer Res* 1999;19:1375–1382.

Shen P, Stewart JH 4th, Levine EA. Cytoreductive surgery and hyperthermic intraperitoneal chemotherapy for peritoneal surface malignancy: overview and rationale. *Curr Probl Cancer* 2009;33:125–141.

Smeenk RM, Bex A, Verwaal VJ, Horenblas S, Zoetmulder FAN. Pseudomyxoma peritonei and the urinary tract: involvement and treatment related complications. *J Surg Oncol* 2006;93:20–23.

Smeenk RM, Verwaal VJ, Antonini N, Zoetmulder FAN. Survival analysis of pseudomyxoma peritonei patients treated by cytoreductive surgery and hyperthermic intraperitoneal chemotherapy. *Ann Surg* 2007;245:104–109.

Sridhar KS, Doria R, Raub W Jr, Thurer RJ, Saldana M. New strategies are needed in diffuse malignant mesothelioma. *Cancer* 1992;70:2969–2979.

Stewart JH 4th, Shen P, Levine EA. Intraperitoneal hyperthermic chemotherapy for peritoneal surface malignancy: current status and future directions. *Ann Surg Oncol* 2005;12:765–777.

Sugarbaker PH. Pseudomyxoma peritonei. A cancer whose biology is characterized by a redistribution phenomenon. *Ann Surg* 1994;219:109–111.

Sugarbaker PH. Peritonectomy procedures. *Ann Surg* 1995;221:29–42.

Sugarbaker PH. Pseudomyxoma peritonei. *Cancer Treat Res* 1996;81:105–119.

Sugarbaker PH, Chang D. Results of treatment of 385 patients with peritoneal surface spread of appendiceal malignancy. *Ann Surg Oncol* 1999;6:727–731.

Sugarbaker PH, Welch LS, Mohamed F, Glehen O. A review of peritoneal mesothelioma at The Washington cancer institute. *Surg Oncol Clin N Am* 2003;12:605–21, xi.

Szych C, Staebler A, Connolly DC, Wu R, Cho KR, Ronnett BM. Molecular genetic evidence supporting the clonality and appendiceal origin of pseudomyxoma peritonei in women. *Am J Pathol* 1999;154:1849–1855.

Van der Speeten K, Stuart OA, Sugarbaker PH. Pharmacokinetics and pharmacodynamics of perioperative cancer chemotherapy in peritoneal surface malignancy. *Cancer J* 2009;15:216–224.

Verwaal VJ, van Ruth S, de Bree E, van Sloothen GW, van Tinteren H, Boot H, Zoetmulder FAN. Randomized trial of cytoreduction and hyperthermic intraperitoneal chemotherapy versus systemic chemotherapy and palliative surgery in patients with peritoneal carcinomatosis of colorectal cancer. *J Clin Oncol* 2003;21:3737–3743.

Verwaal VJ, van Ruth S, Witkamp A, Boot H, van Slooten G, Zoetmulder FAN. Long-term survival of peritoneal carcinomatosis of colorectal origin. *Ann Surg Oncol* 2005;12:65–71.

Vlasveld LT, Gallee MP, Rodenhuis S, Taal BG. Intraperitoneal chemotherapy for malignant peritoneal mesothelioma. *Eur J Cancer* 1991;27:732–734.

Witkamp AJ, de Bree E, Kaag MM, Boot H, Beijnen JH, van Slooten GW, van Coevorden F, Zoetmulder FA. Extensive cytoreductive surgery followed by intra-operative hyperthermic intraperitoneal chemotherapy with mitomycin-c in patients with peritoneal carcinomatosis of colorectal origin. *Eur J Cancer* 2001;37:979–984.

Yan TD, Brun EA, Cerruto CA, Haveric N, Chang D, Sugarbaker PH. Prognostic indicators for patients undergoing cytoreductive surgery and perioperative intraperitoneal chemotherapy for diffuse malignant peritoneal mesothelioma. *Ann Surg Oncol* 2007;14:41–49.

Yan TD, Links M, Xu ZY, Kam PC, Glenn D, Morris DL. Cytoreductive surgery and perioperative intraperitoneal chemotherapy for pseudomyxoma peritonei from appendiceal mucinous neoplasms. *Br J Surg* 2006;93:1270–1276.

Yan TD, Morris DL. Cytoreductive surgery and perioperative intraperitoneal chemotherapy for isolated colorectal peritoneal carcinomatosis: experimental therapy or standard of care? *Ann Surg* 2008;248:829–835.

Yancik R. Ovarian cancer. Age contrasts in incidence, histology, disease stage at diagnosis, and mortality. *Cancer* 1993;71:517–523.

Yates DH, Corrin B, Stidolph PN, Browne K. Malignant mesothelioma in south east England: clinicopathological experience of 272 cases. *Thorax* 1997;52:507–512.

Yonemura Y, de Aretxabala X, Fujimura T, Fushida S, Katayama K, Bandou E, Sugiyama K, Kawamura T, Kinoshita K, Endou Y, Sasaki T. Intraoperative chemohyperthermic peritoneal perfusion as an adjuvant to gastric cancer: final results of a randomized controlled study. *Hepatogastroenterology* 2001;48:1776–1782.

Yonemura Y, Fujimura T, Nishimura G, FallaR, Sawa T, Katayama K, Tsugawa K, Fushida S, Miyazaki I, Tanaka M, Endou Y, Sasaki T. Effects of intraoperative chemohyperthermia in patients with gastric cancer with peritoneal dissemination. *Surgery* 1996;119:437–444.